Sports Nutrition for the Child Athlete

Debbi Sowell Jennings, MS, RD

Pediatric Nutrition Practice Group of
    The American Dietetic Association

Department of Pediatrics

University of Alabama at Birmingham

Birmingham, Alabama

Suzanne Nelson Steen, DSc, RD

Sports and Cardiovascular Nutritionists Practice Group of
    The American Dietetic Association

Department of Clinical Nutrition

The Children's Hospital of Philadelphia

Philadelphia, Pennsylvania

The American Dietetic Association

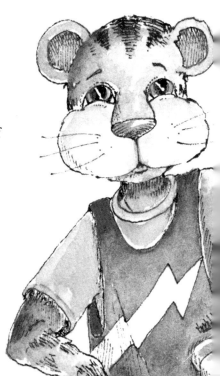

Library of Congress Cataloging-in-Publication Data

Jennings, Debbi Sowell.
    Sports nutrition for the child athlete / Debbi Sowell
Jennings, Suzanne Nelson Steen.
        p.   cm.
    ISBN 0-88091-114-X
    1. Sports for children–Physiological aspects. 2.
Children–Nutrition. I. Steen, Suzanne Nelson. II. Title.
    RC1218.C45J46 1993
    613.2'08'8796–dc20   93-23145

The views represented in this publication are those of the authors and do not necessarily reflect policies and/or official positions of The American Dietetic Association. Mention of product names in this publication does not constitute endorsement by the authors or The American Dietetic Association. The American Dietetic Association disclaims responsibility for the application of the information contained herein.

◆◆◆

Contributors

Jacqueline R. Berning, MS, RD

Ginny B. Kisler, MS, RD

Barbara H. Lummis, MS, RD

Josephine Connolly Schoonen, MS, RD

Maria H. Seman, MS, RD

Laura B. Szekely, MS, RD

DeAnn Whitmire, MS, RD

Reviewers

M.T. DiFerante, MPH, RD

Alice Lindeman, PhD, RD

Lori Valencic, MEd, RD

Nancy Wooldridge, MS, RD

Technical Editor

Michelle L. Kienholz

Artist

Robin M.N. Richards

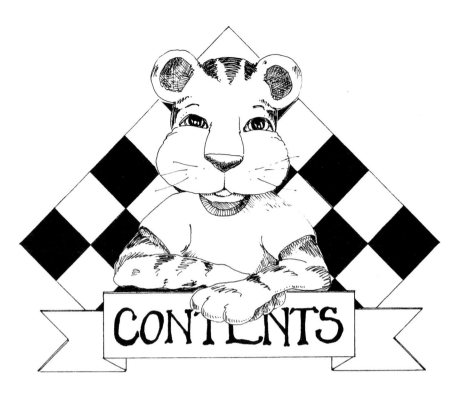

CONTENTS

♦♦

Introduction

As health professionals encourage America's children to become more physically active, and as childhood sports become more competitive, the topic of sports nutrition surfaces more often. This publication, *Sports Nutrition for the Child Athlete*, addresses common concerns of coaches and parents regarding the nutrition needs of exercising children aged 6 to 12 years.

Children, whether athletes or nonathletes, have dietary requirements that are different from those of adults. This book reviews these requirements together with issues of growth, development, and body composition. In addition to the basics, the roles of specific nutrients are discussed, particularly the macronutrients: carbohydrate, protein, and fat. Other topics include fluids, vitamins, and minerals. Practical advice is given on precompetition and postcompetition meals, training diets, and selecting appropriate foods while traveling. Finally, more serious issues that have become increasingly prevalent in the United States, such as eating disorders and proper methods of weight management, are addressed.

In addition to the clear explanations and advice given throughout the book, each chapter is summarized in reproducible handout materials located in the back of this book. The front of each handout is designed in a question-answer format for use by parents or coaches and includes food ideas, menus, recipes, and so forth. The back is designed as a game to help children learn about various nutrition topics.

Before beginning the book, please take a moment to review *Table 1*. Child athletes have the right to enjoy their activities and to strive for success. They cannot do so if they are told fallacies or have already formed wrong ideas about how much and what to eat before, during, and after exercise. The information in this book will help ensure that young athletes are guaranteed these rights with regard to proper nutrition in training and competition.

Table 1. Young Athlete's Bill of Rights

1   The right to have the opportunity to participate in sports regardless of ability level.

2   The right to participate at a level commensurate with the child's developmental level.

3   The right to have qualified adult leadership.

4   The right to participate in a safe and healthy environment.

5   The right of each child to share leadership and decision-making.

6   The right to play as a child and not as an adult.

7   The right to proper preparation for participation in sports.

8   The right to equal opportunity to strive for success.

9   The right to be treated with dignity by all involved.

10   The right to have fun through sports.

Am J Dis Child 1988; 142:143. © 1988 AMA. Reprinted with permission from the American Medical Association.

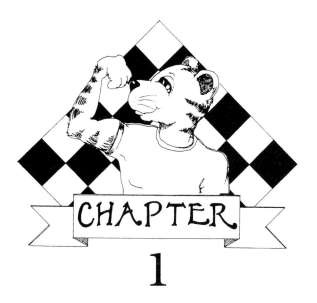

CHAPTER 1

The Growing Child Athlete

Many coaches and parents have questions about the growth and development of their young athletes, such as:

◆ Should 7-year-old boys and girls play soccer together?

◆ Can my 8-year-old son increase muscle by weight lifting?

◆ Should my 11-year-old premenstrual daughter try to reduce her body fat?

◆ How much should my 6-year-old weigh?

This chapter answers these and other questions that you might have. You should be sure that your school-age athletes are growing "on schedule" and that they are eating the right types and amounts of food for their age group.

You might also need to be careful about how you look at any young "superstars." You probably know the importance of body composition—the amount of body fat and muscle mass—in adult athletes. However, because children grow in rapid but somewhat unpredictable spurts, you cannot use ordinary methods for measuring body composition in developing children. Their body chemistry, bone density, and proportion of body water are all significantly different from those of mature athletes, even if their physical performance seems well beyond their years.

Physical Growth

From age 2 until puberty (when children begin to mature sexually), boys and girls grow at about the same rate. You should expect children to grow 2 to 3 inches and gain 3 to 6 pounds each year. There is no *physical* reason to assign young children to single-sex athletic teams. In fact, many organized sports combine girls and boys in group athletics until age 9 or 10, after which they are separated for social reasons.

At puberty, however, children undergo hormonal changes that mark the beginning of adolescence. These hormonal changes cause them to grow rapidly; therefore, you need to watch children entering puberty very carefully to ensure that they are meeting their nutrition needs. Both boys and girls gain body fat just prior to their growth spurt. By storing extra fat, the body has enough calories to fuel the rapid change in height. You should explain this in advance to growing children so they do not hurt their bodies or stunt their growth by trying to imitate the dieting practices of adult athletes.

To help you monitor maturing athletes, a numerical system has been established for describing children in terms of how their bodies are physically changing and developing sexually. This system is known as the Tanner stages of development or Sexual Maturity Ratings (SMR, *Table 1.1*).

Table 1.1. Tanner Stages of Development

Stage	Boys	Girls
1	Prepubescent	Prepubescent
2	First appearance of pubic hair	First appearance of pubic hair
	Growth of genitalia	Development of genitalia
	Increased activity of sweat glands	Increased activity of sweat glands
3	Pubic hair extends to scrotum	Pubic hair thicker, coarser, curly
	Growth and pigmentation of genitalia	Breasts enlarge and pigmentation continues
	Changes in voice	Genitalia well developed
	Beginning of acne	Beginning of acne
4	Pubic hair thickens, facial hair begins	Pubic hair abundant, armpit hair begins
	Growth and pigmentation of genitalia	Breasts enlarge and mature
	Voice deepens	Genitalia assume adult structure
	Acne may be severe	Acne may be severe
		Menarche begins
5	Increased distribution of hair	Increased pubic hair distribution
	Genitalia fully mature	Breasts fully mature
	Acne may persist and increase	Increased severity of acne (if present)

Peak growth spurt in girls

Peak growth spurt in boys

Although formal Tanner staging is measured by a physician, other characteristics can be used to estimate the level of sexual maturity. For girls, knowledge of when menstruation begins is a good rule of thumb to follow. Between Tanner stages 2 and 3 (usually ages 11 to 12 in the United States), girls undergo their peak growth spurt, with an average gain of 3.25 inches in height. Menstruation begins at stage 4. Once a girl has begins menses, the rapid period of growth is completed.

Boys grow fastest between Tanner stages 3 and 4 (usually between ages 13 and 14). Boys can expect to grow 8 inches during this phase. Following the growth spurt (in Tanner stage 4), the boy has enough circulating male hormones in the blood to add muscle mass and to show signs of facial hair. If a boy has only "peach fuzz" for facial hair, he may not have completed his growth spurt. The growth spurt lasts much longer in boys than in girls, and after the growth spurt, boys continue to grow at a slow pace until approximately age 20.

Strength

Girls and boys have about the same strength until puberty. Girls gain strength as they grow until they start to menstruate, whereas boys continue to become stronger after they finish their growth spurt. After puberty, boys are generally stronger than girls.

By using the Tanner staging system, you can estimate the athletic capabilities of children and teens so that boys and girls are fairly matched and trained properly. For example:

- A 10-year-old tennis player would benefit very little from a weight-lifting program due to the lack of circulating androgens, which are male hormones necessary for muscle development.

- A 12-year-old basketball player who has not begun menses might be encouraged by the fact that her growth spurt has not ended.

- An 11-year-old premenstrual girl should not diet to reduce body fat, which the body stores just prior to menarche.

Body Measurements

You probably know that height/weight status in children is checked against national growth standards prepared by the National Center of Health Statistics. Pediatricians and registered dietitians regularly use these charts to assess children's height and weight up to age 18. If you have any questions about the normal growth of any athlete, you should refer him or her to a pediatrician and a registered dietitian.

You also may have read about measuring body fat in adult athletes. This practice has become popular in schools and training rooms as well. Common techniques for measuring body fat include underwater weighing (a complicated and expensive technique in which the athlete is submerged in a water tank), bioelectrical impedance (or BIA, another expensive technique that is valid only when used with well-hydrated athletes), and skinfold measurements with calipers, such as the Lange or the Harpenden models (a technique that must be performed by a well-trained professional). However, methods for measuring fat are limited in children due to changes in the body that occur before they mature and as they mature. Even trained exercise physiologists have difficulty accurately estimating the percentage of body fat in children and must use special mathematical equations. An untrained person who is not familiar with these equations probably will overestimate body fat in children and may underestimate lean body weight, leading to an inappropriate or unsafe weight goal.

> **Body fat measurements should *never* be used to manipulate any child's weight for sports competition or to set weight management guidelines.**
> **The normal growth and development of the child athlete always must be the primary concern.**

Dietary Recommendations

What should young athletes eat? The US Department of Agriculture and Department of Health and Human Services publish the *Dietary Guidelines,* which recommend a healthful way for all Americans to eat. The Guidelines call for moderation and variety in the diet.

- Eat a variety of foods.
- Maintain a healthy weight.
- Choose a diet low in fat, saturated fat, and cholesterol.
- Choose a diet with plenty of vegetables, fruits, and grain products.
- Use sugars only in moderation.
- Use salt and sodium only in moderation.
- If you drink alcoholic beverages, do so in moderation.

To understand what these guidelines really mean in a child's diet, let us look at the Food Guide Pyramid *(Figure 1.1)*, which was developed by the US Department of Agriculture as a visual guide for planning healthful meals. Each section of the pyramid represents a food category and gives a range for the number of recommended servings to be consumed daily *(Tables 1.2 and 1.3)*. Generally, providing servings within this range will supply the necessary nutrients and energy most active children need.

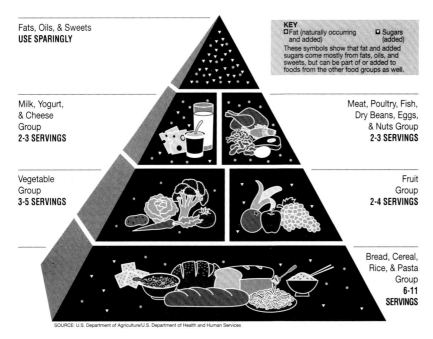

Fats, Oils, & Sweets
USE SPARINGLY

KEY
▫ Fat (naturally occurring and added)   ▪ Sugars (added)
These symbols show that fat and added sugars come mostly from fats, oils, and sweets, but can be part of or added to foods from the other food groups as well.

Milk, Yogurt, & Cheese Group
2-3 SERVINGS

Meat, Poultry, Fish, Dry Beans, Eggs, & Nuts Group
2-3 SERVINGS

Vegetable Group
3-5 SERVINGS

Fruit Group
2-4 SERVINGS

Bread, Cereal, Rice, & Pasta Group
6-11 SERVINGS

SOURCE: U.S. Department of Agriculture/U.S. Department of Health and Human Services

Figure 1.1. The Food Guide Pyramid: a guide to daily food choices.

Table 1.2. How Many Servings of Each Food Group Does the Active Child Need Each Day?

Food Group	No. of Servings
Bread	9
Vegetable	4
Fruit	3
Milk	2-3
Meat	2-3

(Total grams of fat = 73)

Caloric level is about 2200. The exercising child may need an additional 500 to 1500 Calories each day, depending on the frequency, intensity, and duration of physical activity.

You can help determine whether a child is eating enough calories by tracking his or her height and weight and comparing them with national growth standards. You also should watch how well a child performs and ask whether he or she is tired or "out of steam." If so, he or she may not be eating enough. Of course, a pediatrician or registered dietitian must decide whether the child's diet needs to be changed. If a health professional makes recommendations for weight gain or weight loss, read chapter 9 for general guidelines.

But before you or anyone else can make any dietary recommendations, examine the actual diet of the young athlete. Measuring exactly what children eat is difficult, but a registered dietitian can estimate the amounts of calories, protein, carbohydrate, fat, and vitamins and minerals that are eaten on a regular basis. If you are ever concerned about the adequacy of a child's diet, consult a registered dietitian to identify any problems that may be hindering performance.

Table 1.3. How Big Is a Serving?

Group	Examples
Bread	1 slice of bread or $\frac{1}{2}$ bun or bagel 1 ounce of ready-to-eat cereal $\frac{1}{2}$ cup of cooked cereal, rice, or pasta
Vegetable	1 cup of raw, leafy vegetables $\frac{1}{2}$ cup of chopped, cooked or canned vegetables $\frac{3}{4}$ cup of vegetable juice
Fruit	1 medium apple, banana, orange $\frac{1}{2}$ cup of cooked or canned fruit $\frac{3}{4}$ cup of pure fruit juice
Milk	1 cup of milk or yogurt $1\frac{1}{2}$ ounce of natural cheese 2 ounces of processed cheese
Meat	2–3 ounces of cooked, lean meat, poultry, or fish $\frac{1}{2}$ cup cooked dry beans or 1 egg 2 tablespoons of peanut butter

The most common tools for assessing dietary intake include food records, 24-hour food recalls, and food frequency forms. Information recorded on a typical food record includes:

- the type or brand of food;
- the amount of food eaten;
- the time at which each food was eaten; and
- the manner in which the food was cooked and/or prepared (including toppings).

Any side effects the food may have had on the athlete during exercise also should be recorded. For example, keeping food records may help a rising track star understand that breakfast cannot be skipped too often, that potato chips eaten before practice do not settle well, or that ice cream eaten in the evening should give way to low-fat frozen yogurt.

Summary

When planning nutrition for a growing athlete, consider the child as well as the sport. You can use his or her stage of growth and development to predict nutrition needs and physical capabilities. Remember, too, that children look up to coaches, trainers, teachers, and parents as role models. If you set a good example by exercising and eating a nourishing, balanced diet, a child athlete is more likely to "eat to compete" and thereby grow into a healthy adult.

CHAPTER

2

Carbohydrate

Young, growing athletes work hard, play hard, and place extra demands on their bodies as a result. Proper training combined with sound nutrition practices can help child athletes meet these demands and learn healthy habits for the rest of their lives. However, most children (and adults) neglect nutrition as a key component of good health and athletic performance. Children, especially in the prepubescent years, often skip breakfast and tend to eat the same foods day after day. These habits leave important nutrients out of their diets and may impair growth and athletic performance. Child athletes often need to eat extra calories (see chapter 1), which should be given mainly as carbohydrate foods. This chapter discusses carbohydrate as the preferred fuel for exercise, including the types, sources, and dietary recommendations.

Types of Carbohydrate

Carbohydrate foods, or "carbos," are recognized as the cornerstone of the athlete's diet *(Table 2.1)*. Carbohydrate comes mainly from plant foods in two forms: simple and complex.

♦ *Simple* carbohydrate or simple sugar is sweet. It is easily digested and absorbed into the bloodstream to provide quick energy. Simple carbohydrate is found in milk, fruits, and sugary products (candy, cookies, soda).

♦ *Complex* carbohydrate is starchy. Starches found in vegetables like potatoes and corn are examples. They provide energy more slowly because they take longer to be digested into sugar and to be absorbed into the bloodstream as glucose. Complex carbohydrate is found in breads, cereals, pasta, rice, and other starchy foods.

Table 2.1. Which Is Better?

- Both simple and complex carbohydrates provide energy to working muscles.

- Foods that are high in complex carbohydrate contain more essential nutrients, such as B vitamins, iron, dietary fiber, and minerals.

- Simple carbohydrate, especially from foods such as candy and soft drinks or soda pop, may provide energy during exercise but lack essential vitamins and minerals.

- Most carbohydrate in the diet should be obtained from complex carbohydrate food sources.

Carbohydrate in Exercise

After the body digests carbohydrate, it uses it to provide energy. For immediate energy, carbohydrate is turned into glucose, which is circulated in the blood. The liver and muscles can store carbohydrate as glycogen, which can be used for energy (as glucose) later during exercise.

Carbohydrate is used mainly to provide energy for the muscles to do work. How much and what type of fuel (glucose or fat) is used depends on how intense the activity is and how long the exercise lasts.

- Brief, intense exercise, such as sprinting or weight lifting, uses glucose from glycogen stored in the muscles for fuel.

- Intermittent sports, such as basketball or football, also use glucose from stored glycogen for fuel.

- Endurance sports, such as long-distance running or cycling, use glycogen stores first and then turn to body fat (see chapter 4) for energy.

- For any activity, the body prefers to use carbohydrate for energy.

However, the muscles and liver can store only a limited amount of glycogen. Glycogen must be replaced by eating more carbohydrate, especially after exercise. Child athletes who experience fatigue or sluggishness might be training too hard, might be dehydrated, might be eating too little, or might be eating too little carbohydrate. Active children should eat at least 50% to 55% of their total calories in the form of carbohydrate.

Dietary Recommendations

Young athletes should think of carbohydrate when they think about food. For example, the school-aged child athlete who needs to eat 2500 Calories per day would need to eat at least 313 to 343 grams of carbohydrate (there are 4 Calories per gram of carbohydrate). Foods that have high levels of complex carbohydrate, such as potatoes, rice, cereals, and starchy vegetables, are excellent sources of glucose as well. Fruits, fruit juices, and dairy products contain natural simple sugars. Review the list of high-carbohydrate foods in *Table 2.2* to make suggestions to your young athletes.

Table 2.2. High-Carbohydrate Foods

Food Group	Serving	*Energy (Calories)*	*Carbohydrates (grams)*
Bread, Cereal, Rice, and Pasta— These foods provide a higher percentage of complex carbohydrate.			
Rice (brown)	1 cup cooked	232	50
Rice (white)	1 cup cooked	223	50
Noodles (spaghetti)	1 cup cooked	159	34
Bagel	1	165	31
English muffin	1	154	30
Corn bread (2-in square)	1	178	28
Oatmeal (flavored instant)	1 packet	110	25
Cereal (cold, ready-to-eat)	1 cup	110	24
Pretzels	1 ounce	106	21
Bun (hot dog, hamburger)	1	119	21
Cereal (cooked, cream of wheat)	¾ cup	96	19
Pancakes (4-in across)	2	112	18
Waffles (3.5-in across)	2	120	17
Blueberry muffin	1	110	17
Tortilla (flour)	1	85	15
Bread sticks	2 sticks	77	15
Biscuit (2-in across)	1	103	13
Oatmeal (cooked)	½ cup	66	12
Bread (white, whole-wheat)	1 slice	61	12
Graham crackers	2 squares	60	11
Saltines	5 crackers	60	10
Popcorn (plain)	1 cup popped	26	6

continued

Table 2.2. High-Carbohydrate Foods *(continued)*

Food Group	Serving	Energy (Calories)	Carbohydrates (grams)
Other baked goods— **These foods provide both complex and simple carbohydrate.**			
Chocolate cake	1 piece	235	40
Angel food cake	1 piece	142	32
Granola bar	1	109	16
Animal crackers	5	56	10
Fig bar	1	50	10
Oatmeal raisin cookie	1	62	9
Combination foods— **These foods provide a higher percentage of complex carbohydrate.**			
Pizza (cheese)	1 slice	290	39
Bean burrito	1	393	32
Fruit— **These foods provide a higher percentage of simple carbohydrate.**			
Raisins (seedless)	²/₃ cup	302	79
Dates (dried)	10	228	61
Applesauce	1 cup	232	60
Prunes (dried)	10	201	53
Grapes	1 cup	147	37
Apple juice	1 cup	111	28
Banana	1	105	27
Orange juice	1 cup	112	26
Grape juice	1 cup	96	23
Apple	1 medium	81	21
Pineapple	1 cup	77	19
Pear	1	77	19
Orange	1 medium	65	16
Fruit cocktail (packed in own juice)	½ cup	56	15
Raspberries	1 cup	61	14
Cantaloupe	1 cup	57	14
Watermelon	1 cup	50	12
Cherries (raw)	10	49	11
Strawberries	1 cup	45	11
Vegetable— **These foods provide a higher percentage of complex carbohydrate.**			
Potato (baked, plain)	1 large	220	50
Lima beans	1 cup cooked	217	39

Food Group	Serving	Energy (Calories)	Carbohydrates (grams)
Sweet potato	1 large	118	28
Corn	½ cup	89	21
Peas (green)	½ cup	63	12
Carrot	1 medium	31	8
Milk, Yogurt, and Cheese— **These foods provide a higher percentage of simple** **carbohydrate.**			
Fruit-flavored yogurt	1 cup	225	42
Frozen yogurt (low-fat)	1 cup	220	34
Pudding (any flavor)	½ cup	161	30
Milk (1%)	1 cup	121	12
Milk (skim)	1 cup	86	12

Depending on their caloric needs, school-age child athletes can add more carbohydrate to their diets by eating at least the following amounts from the Food Guide Pyramid groups (*Figure 2.1*):

- ◆ Six servings from the Bread, Cereal, Rice, and Pasta group
- ◆ Three servings from the Milk, Yogurt, and Cheese group
- ◆ Three servings from the Vegetable group
- ◆ Two servings from the Fruit group

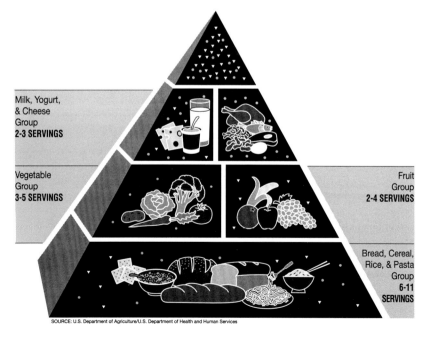

SOURCE: U.S. Department of Agriculture/U.S. Department of Health and Human Services

Figure 2.1. The Food Guide Pyramid: carbohydrate food groups.

You can help children remember which foods to choose by putting them on "teams" as shown in *Table 2.3*. Ask your team members to pick winning carbohydrates from each team to eat.

Table 2.3. Winning Carbohydrates

Bread, Cereal, Rice, and Pasta Team	Fruit and Vegetable Team	Milk, Yogurt, and Cheese Team
Bagel	Apples	Milk
Breads	Bananas	Yogurt
Cereals	Broccoli	Pudding
Crackers	Corn	Frozen yogurt
English muffins	Carrots	Sherbet
Graham crackers	Fruit juices	
Pancakes	Nectarines	
Pasta (spaghetti, macaroni)	Oranges	
	Pears	
Popcorn	Peas	
Potato,	Peppers (green, red)	
sweet potato	Tomatoes	
Pretzels		
Rice		

The sample menu in *Table 2.4* would be appropriate for many young athletes and would provide about 2500 Calories with about 55% of calories from carbohydrate, 15% to 20% from protein, and 25% to 30% from fat.

Trying to provide well-balanced meals and snacks for child athletes can be a challenge. To help children eat more carbohydrate, you can:

- ◆ Encourage them to consume carbohydrate-rich foods at meals and as snacks.

- ◆ Try to include at least one serving each from the Bread, Cereal, Rice, and Pasta group, the Vegetable group, the Fruit group, and the Milk, Yogurt, and Cheese group at each meal. (Two thirds of the food on children's plates should have plenty of carbohydrate!)

- ◆ Pack easy-to-carry carbohydrate foods for lunch and pre-practice snacks: bagels, oatmeal raisin cookies, fruit bars, pretzels, fig bars, low-fat yogurt, popcorn, fresh fruit or juice, pudding, raisins, bananas, and so forth.

- ◆ Let young athletes have a "refreshment" break during practice to drink fluids and to eat carbohydrate-rich snacks.

- ◆ Correct poor eating habits gradually by including more nutritious foods.

- ◆ Encourage children to help make their own meals and snacks.

- ◆ Serve children's favorite foods along with nutritious, high-carbohydrate, low-fat foods.

Table 2.4. Sample Menu

Meal	Menu
Breakfast	2 pancakes Syrup 1 cup 2% milk
Snack	1 bagel Jam or jelly 6 ounces orange juice
Lunch	1 slice vegetable pizza Carrot and celery sticks 2 graham crackers 1 cup 2% milk
Snack	*Before practice:* 2 fig bars 16 ounces water *After practice:* 1 box fruit juice 1 packet raisins
Dinner	3 ounces roasted chicken breast $\frac{1}{2}$ cup broccoli $\frac{1}{2}$ cup rice 1 slice bread Lettuce and tomato 1 tablespoon dressing 1 cup 2% milk
Snack	1 cup frozen yogurt 1 cup lemonade 1 sandwich (2 slices multigrain bread, 3 ounces lean turkey, lettuce and tomato, mustard)

Summary

In general, school-age child athletes need more energy to fuel both their exercise and normal growth and development. Eating carbohydrate allows the muscles to store glycogen for fuel during exercise. Children who do not eat enough carbohydrate may not train or compete up to par. You should encourage all school-age children—particularly child athletes—to eat more carbohydrate foods and to replace high-fat items, such as snack chips, ice cream, and pastries, with more healthful, high-carbohydrate foods, such as breads, corn, fruits, and spaghetti.

CHAPTER

3

Protein

Protein is an essential part of child athletes' diets . . . as long as it is eaten in moderation. The role of protein in sports nutrition has reached mythical proportions that must be reduced to reality. What is the real story? The following common questions regarding protein are answered in this chapter:

- ◆ How does the body use protein?
- ◆ Will extra protein improve athletic performance?
- ◆ How much protein does the child athlete need?

Athletes can adjust the amount of protein they eat for optimal performance in training and in competition, but protein and amino acids (which make up protein) have no magical qualities that guarantee success. Protein alone cannot and will not improve athletic ability, no matter what manufacturers of special amino acid supplements would have the public believe. This chapter addresses dietary protein and protein requirements for young athletes.

Protein in the Body

Protein is one of the basic nutrients found in most foods. It is made from building blocks called *amino acids*. Although some advertisements suggest that certain amino acids build muscle, amino acids actually build protein that the body uses in many different ways. Despite the many claims for using protein to boost athletic performance, the main function of protein is to maintain and repair all body tissues. Protein also makes:

- ◆ hemoglobin, which takes oxygen to all cells.
- ◆ antibodies, which fight off infection and disease.
- ◆ enzymes and hormones, which regulate body functions.

Eating extra protein does not improve any of these functions, and it does not make stronger or larger muscles. Extra protein is usually stored as fat, not as muscle, so eating too much protein can sometimes hurt the body more than it helps it.

Building Muscles

While protein is used by the body to make muscle tissue, eating large amounts of protein does not lead to the development of larger, stronger muscles. Muscles do not get bigger unless the body has enough male hormones (androgens) in the blood (see chapter 1). Boys and girls both add muscle during the pubertal process, but boys eventually have more androgens circulating in the bloodstream, which result in greater muscle mass. Even these androgens do not magically build muscles. To gain muscle mass, athletes must increase the workload on their muscles (with training) and eat a balanced diet.

How Much Protein Should Young Athletes Eat?

Although the Recommended Dietary Allowances (RDAs) tell how much protein boys and girls should eat at different ages *(Table 3.1)*, other factors should be considered:

- ◆ **Maturity**—Young athletes who are at or beyond the stage of sexual maturity at which they can add muscle mass because they have the proper hormones may have slightly higher protein needs (see chapter 1 for discussion of the maturation process).

- ◆ **Carbohydrates**—Although it is *not* recommended, young athletes who eat little carbohydrate may need slightly more protein; children who eat the recommended high-carbohydrate diet should need only the recommended amount of protein for their age and gender.

- ◆ **Calories**—Young athletes who eat too few calories may need slightly more protein, but the best idea would be to increase overall food intake.

- ◆ **Training**—Young athletes who follow hard, exhausting training schedules may need more protein, but only temporarily during the training season.

- ◆ **Protein sources**—Young athletes who eat most or all of their proteins from plant sources must be careful to eat a wide variety of grains and vegetables, while children who eat proteins from a variety of animal sources (meat, milk, eggs) usually do not have to worry about getting enough protein.

Most children 6 to 10 years old need to eat about 0.5 gram of protein per pound of body weight each day. Young athletes who might need slightly more protein (for reasons previously described) can eat 0.6 to 0.9 gram of protein per pound of body weight. You should realize, though, that this additional amount of protein is supplied in just an extra glass of milk or an extra serving of meat (3 to 4 ounces).

Table 3.1. RDAs for Protein

Age (years), Gender	Daily Protein Intake (grams)
4–6, all	24
7–10, all	28
11–14, boys	45
15–18, boys	59
11–14, girls	46
15–18, girls	44

For example, your 10-year-old soccer player should eat about 0.5 gram of protein per pound of body weight. If he weighs 70 pounds, he should eat about 35 grams of protein per day. If for any of the reasons discussed he needs slightly more protein, he should not eat more than 0.6 to 0.9 gram of protein per pound of body weight per day. The 70-pound soccer player therefore should not eat more than 42 to 63 grams of protein per day, even during rigorous training. The next section will help you estimate how much protein is in the different foods that children usually eat.

Protein in Foods

Young athletes can easily meet their protein needs on a diet that includes at least the following amounts of foods recommended in the Food Guide Pyramid *(Figure 3.1)*:

- Two to three servings of meat, poultry, fish, dry beans and peas, eggs, nuts
- Three servings of low-fat milk, yogurt, cheese
- Six servings of bread, cereal, rice, pasta
- Three servings of vegetables

Young athletes should spread their protein choices throughout the day rather than having one large serving of protein-rich food in the evening. They also should eat a variety of protein foods from each of the food groups *(Table 3.2)*.

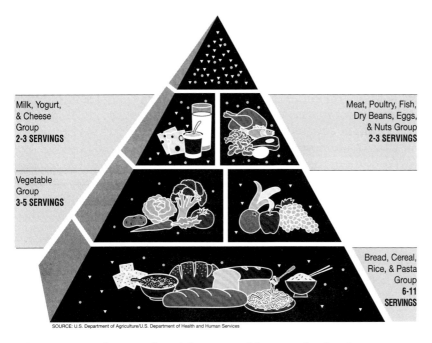

Milk, Yogurt,
& Cheese
Group
2-3 SERVINGS

Meat, Poultry, Fish,
Dry Beans, Eggs,
& Nuts Group
2-3 SERVINGS

Vegetable
Group
3-5 SERVINGS

Bread, Cereal,
Rice, & Pasta
Group
**6-11
SERVINGS**

SOURCE: U.S. Department of Agriculture/U.S. Department of Health and Human Services

Figure 3.1. The Food Guide Pyramid: protein food groups.

Table 3.2. Protein in Various Foods

Food	Protein (grams)	Serving Size
Milk	8	8 ounces (1 cup)
Yogurt	8	8 ounces (1 cup)
Cheese	7	1 ounce (1 slice or cube)
Fish	21	3 ounces (tuna sandwich)
Poultry	21	3 ounces (grilled chicken sandwich)
Meat (beef)	21	3 ounces (hamburger, roast beef sandwich)
Peanut butter	4	1 tablespoon
Nuts	5–7	1 ounce (1 handful)
Eggs	7	1

What About Protein Supplements?

Protein, whether from food or dietary supplements, is made up of amino acids. Some of the amino acids can be made in the body, and others cannot. The ones that are made in the body are called *nonessential amino acids.* The ones that are not made in the body are called *essential amino acids* and must be eaten in the diet. Of the 22 amino acids, 13 are nonessential and nine are essential.

If you think that any of your young players may need any type of nutritional supplement, please reconsider. One of the dangers of eating too much protein is dehydration. Protein and amino acid supplements are especially unnecessary in children, since most supplements are expensive and do not contain any more protein or amino acids than are found in a serving of meat or a glass of milk. The body treats amino acids from powders the same way as it does amino acids from oat ring cereal. Consider *Table 3.3.*

Table 3.3. Amino Acids Provided in Food Source Versus Supplement

Amino Acid	Quantity (milligrams) in Cereal (1 oz) + Milk (½ cup)	Quantity (milligrams) in Amino Acid Supplement*
Threonine (essential)	329	24
Isoleucine (essential)	588	40
Lysine (essential)	492	135
Methionine (essential)	171	20
Cysteine (nonessential)	144	0
Phenylalanine (essential)	425	280
Tyrosine (nonessential)	346	8
Valine (essential)	519	38
Arginine (nonessential)	465	1000
Histidine (essential)	205	0

*This is an average "amino acid package."

No individual or group of amino acids will improve athletic performance or muscle bulk or strength.

Vegetarian Diet

When discussing how much protein to eat, it is generally assumed that the athlete will be consuming a variety of foods from all food groups—meat, milk, bread, vegetable, and fruit. Animal foods—such as eggs, milk, yogurt, cheese, fish, poultry, beef, and pork—contain proteins that include all the essential amino acids. Proteins found in plant products (vegetables and grains) are "incomplete," meaning that they do not contain all nine essential amino acids. Therefore, vegetarian athletes must eat a wide variety of plant proteins to ensure a combination of all essential amino acids. Plant foods that lack one or more amino acids can be eaten with other plant foods that are rich in the missing amino acid(s). *Table 3.4* shows examples of how plant foods can be eaten together to provide all the essential amino acids.

Table 3.4. Plant Food Combinations Yielding All Essential Amino Acids

Rice + beans (kidney, pinto, lima, navy)

Croutons + split-pea soup

Tortillas + beans

Corn bread + chili beans

Brown bread + baked beans

Whole-wheat bread + peanut butter

Tofu + sesame seeds

Any of your young athletes who follows a vegetarian diet must be careful of what he or she eats. The vegetarian diet can be nutritionally complete so long as a wide variety of foods are consumed over the course of a day. However, any child on a vegetarian diet should be referred to a registered dietitian to check the nutritional adequacy of his or her diet. The dietitian can teach the young athlete and his or her parents about a balanced vegetarian diet and advise them to eat milk foods and eggs to make sure that the child grows properly and can remain physically active.

A vegetarian who does not eat animal flesh, eggs, or milk products may be at risk for nutrient deficiencies of:

◆ Vitamin B_{12}—found reliably only in animal sources and in some fortified cereals.

◆ Calcium—best consumed in milk, yogurt, and other dairy products.

◆ Iron—not absorbed as well from plant sources as from animal sources; even a small portion of meat, poultry, or fish with an iron-rich vegetable will enhance iron absorption.

Eliminating foods that contain important vitamins and minerals can be dangerous unless the children and parents are prepared to take on the additional responsibility necessary to maintain good health and proper growth.

Summary

Protein is essential to the overall health, growth, and development of child athletes. It should come from low-fat animal sources and/or from a wide variety of plant foods. High-protein diets are unnecessary for any athlete—especially child athletes—since most Americans usually consume more protein than their bodies need. Eating excessive amounts of protein burdens the body and is merely stored as fat. Unfortunately, athletes of all ages continue to use protein and amino acid pills, powders, and drinks in the vain hope of increasing muscle mass and strength. Remember, the advertisements for "body-building" supplements promote false hopes of increasing muscle mass when the only actual increase is in the companies' commercial profits!

CHAPTER

4

Fat

A certain amount of body fat is essential to maintain normal body functions. In children whose weights are in the normal range, as discussed in chapter 1, dieting to gain or lose body fat is strongly discouraged because of the dramatic effects it can have on the body during critical stages of growth. Body fat comes mainly from dietary fat, though excessive amounts of protein and carbohydrate can be stored as fat as well. This chapter provides guidelines for how much dietary fat exercising children should eat and discusses the amount of fat in various foods.

Fat in the Body

Fats and oils are essential nutrients in the human diet. Dietary fat (such as margarine or oil) can be added to foods to enhance flavor, encouraging finicky eaters to eat a wider variety of foods. For example, adding margarine to corn may improve the taste so that many children who might not eat it otherwise can enjoy it. When eaten in moderation, fat in food can be a concentrated source of energy for athletes. Fat in the diet:

- supplies more than twice as much energy as protein and carbohydrate (9 Calories per gram of fat, 4 Calories per gram of carbohydrate or protein).
- helps the body absorb and use certain vitamins (A, D, E, and K, which are fat-soluble vitamins).
- supplies essential fatty acids that the body needs to survive.

Body fat stores are found beneath the skin, around the organs, and inside the muscles. Fat is sometimes used as a fuel by muscles in the form of triglycerides, which are present in food and are also made in the liver and intestines. Triglycerides are made of fatty acids (individual fat units) that determine whether fat is saturated, polyunsaturated, or monounsaturated. Saturated fats (such as butter or beef fat) are more unhealthful, particularly for the heart, than unsaturated fats (such as safflower and corn oil) and monounsaturated fats (such as olive and peanut oil).

Fat in Exercise

As discussed in chapter 2, blood sugar and muscle glycogen give working muscles most of their energy. The following factors determine how much fat the body uses for energy.

- ◆ **Duration**—Fat tissue is used to provide energy, but exercise must be performed for 30 minutes before enough fatty acids are available for fuel. Until then, most of the energy is provided by carbohydrate (glycogen).

- ◆ **Intensity**—As the intensity of the exercise increases, working muscles have less oxygen available to burn fat. During sports that have short bouts of very intense activity, such as a 200-yard dash, a 50-yard swim, or a baseball game, very little fat is burned for energy.

Fat in the Diet

How much fat should your young athletes eat? Fat stores play an important role in athletic performance, and fat is an essential nutrient for a growing child. As emphasized in chapter 1, young athletes must take extra care to eat enough calories, protein, and essential vitamins and minerals so that their growth is not affected by the added stress and rigor of athletic activity. When helping young athletes plan their meals, you must consider the recommended percentage of calories from fat, safe levels of cholesterol, and preferred food sources.

The typical American diet supplies 40% of total calories as fat, a figure that is too high and may be responsible for the high incidence of many chronic diseases (such as heart disease, cancer, and diabetes). The American Dietetic Association, the American Academy of Pediatrics, the US Department of Health and Human Services' National Cholesterol Education Program, the American Heart Association, and the National Cancer Institute support the following guidelines for fat consumption:

These recommendations do not apply to infants from birth to 2 years of age because of their rapid rate of growth. These children need to eat a higher percentage of fat calories.

- ◆ **Total fat**—No more than 30% of total daily calories
- ◆ **Saturated fat**—Less than 10% of total daily calories
- ◆ **Cholesterol**—Less than 300 milligrams per day

As you can see, the Food Guide Pyramid recommends using fats and oils sparingly in the diet *(Figure 4.1).*

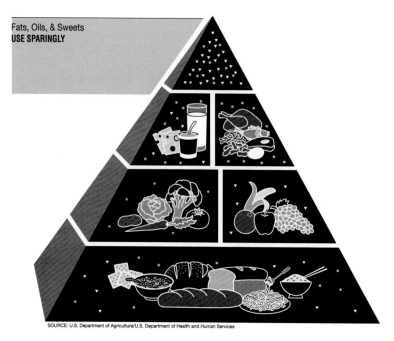

SOURCE: U.S. Department of Agriculture/U.S. Department of Health and Human Services

Figure 4.1. The Food Guide Pyramid: fats, oils, and sweets.

Families should select, prepare, and eat foods that are low in saturated fat, low in total fat, and low in cholesterol. They also should choose a variety of foods to eat enough carbohydrate, protein, and other nutrients while eating only enough calories to maintain desirable body weight.

To reduce the fat in a child's diet, you may want to examine recent food records (see chapter 1) to estimate how many calories the child is eating and to identify the high-fat foods in the diet. Because most food labels provide the fat content in terms of grams, you may find it easier to calculate the number of fat grams that can be eaten each day: divide caloric intake by 30 to determine the number of fat grams that will provide 30% of calories as fat. For example:

- 2000 Calories ÷ 30 = 67 grams of fat (30% of calories)
- 2200 Calories ÷ 30 = 73 grams of fat (30% of calories)
- 2400 Calories ÷ 30 = 80 grams of fat (30% of calories)

Note that this holds true only for 30%. Do not divide by a different number, such as 28, to calculate the number of fat grams for 28% of calories from fat

Most people should be concerned about reducing the amount of fat that they eat. The key to achieving this in child athletes' diets is *moderation*. You should not be too strict *or* too liberal with fat. Taking too much fat out of the diet also can take the fun out of eating. Children, especially physically active children, need a lot of energy and, therefore, need to eat moderate amounts of fat. Of course, children who eat a lot of fried foods, junk foods, desserts, or fast foods (see chapter 8) are probably consuming too much fat that is replacing other essential nutrients.

Cholesterol in the Diet

Cholesterol is found only in animal products. *Usually* foods that have a lot of cholesterol also have a lot of saturated fat—but not always. For example, shellfish (such as shrimp) is very low in saturated fat but relatively high in cholesterol. However, it is always better to select the low-fat shellfish over the high-fat meat. Eating foods that are high in saturated fat raises blood cholesterol levels more than eating foods that are high in cholesterol. The National Cholesterol Education Program recommends that adults as well as healthy children and teens eat no more than 300 milligrams of cholesterol per day.

Summary

The best training diet supplies the athlete's body with all the essential nutrients in the right amounts. Fat is a concentrated source of energy that also makes food taste better. If nutritious foods taste better, the young athlete is more likely to eat nutritionally balanced meals. Severely restricting the amount of fat a child can eat to improve fitness can be dangerous: a critical source of calories is lost, and prolonged fat restriction can have other negative effects on the child's growth and development.

CHAPTER

5

Vitamins and Minerals

In an age of fast foods, frozen entrees for children, sugar-coated breakfast cereals, and candy disguised as fruit products, it is possible for children to eat three meals a day with plenty of calories but few essential nutrients. However, vitamin and mineral supplements are not necessary to ensure adequate nutrient intake. It is easy to give children a well-balanced and *enjoyable* diet of foods readily available in the supermarket. Although preadolescent children may have slower growth rates and reduced appetites, they still must eat enough nutrients to meet minimal dietary requirements and to get ready for their upcoming growth spurt. For young athletes, proper nutrition also promotes optimal athletic performance. Both child athletes and the adults who work with them should be educated on which convenient, nutrient-dense foods can meet daily requirements and improve performance. A wide variety of these foods should be made easily accessible to children both at home and in school. This chapter reviews the functions and sources of essential vitamins and minerals and discusses their role in child athletes' diets.

How Vitamins Help

The body cannot make vitamins on its own and needs to get them through food. Vitamins are essential for life, but some can be reused and, therefore, are needed only in very small amounts each day. The *fat-soluble* vitamins—A, D, E, and K—are stored in the fat tissues of the body. *Water-soluble* vitamins are not stored in the body and must be replaced every day. These include C, thiamin, riboflavin, B_6, niacin, folacin, biotin, and pantothenic acid. *Table 5.1* gives food choices for two important vitamins—A (fat-soluble) and C (water-soluble).

Table 5.1. Food Choices for Vitamins A and C

Vitamin A is important for healthy growth, skin, and vision and is found in:	Vitamin C is important for healthy teeth, bones, and blood vessels and is found in:	Both vitamins A and C are found in:
Asparagus Carrots Collard greens Mixed vegetables Mustard greens Pumpkin Winter squash (acorn, butternut etc)	Brussels sprouts Cauliflower Okra Potatoes	Broccoli Kale Peppers (green, red, chili) Spinach Sweet potatoes Tomatoes Turnip greens
Apricots Cherries (red sour) Nectarines Guavas Prunes	Banana Grapes Grapefruit, grapefruit juice Peaches Honeydew melon	Cantaloupe Mangoes Papayas Plums (purple)
Milk	Lemons Oranges, orange juice Raspberries Strawberries Tangerines Tangelos Watermelon	

Vitamins have many functions in the body. Most of them help the body use carbohydrate, fat, and protein, while others have more specific tasks, such as making red blood cells, regulating growth, clotting blood, and maintaining vision. By keeping the body working properly, vitamins help maintain health and, in children, proper growth and development. However, eating more vitamins or eating them more frequently does not speed up or otherwise help any of the reactions that might be useful to athletic performance *(Table 5.2)*.

Table 5.2. Get the Facts. . .

The best source of vitamins is a healthful, balanced diet.

Vitamins have not been shown to prevent or cure any disease (including the common cold) except for those related to specific vitamin deficiencies (for example, vitamin C cures scurvy).

Although some vitamins help the body produce and use energy, they do not provide energy themselves (because they do not contain any calories).

continued

Table 5.2. Get the Facts. . . *(continued)*

There is no difference between vitamins made in a laboratory and "natural" vitamins from plants or animals (except "natural" vitamins are usually more expensive).

Vitamin supplements *cannot* be used to replace foods or make up for poor dietary habits.

B_{15} (pangamic acid) is not a vitamin.

Taking extra vitamins will not make a child mature faster or become stronger.

Some vitamins are toxic at high doses. "If a little is good, more must be better" does not apply to *any* vitamins.

Minerals in the Body

Minerals are also essential and perform a variety of functions in the body. Some are used to make specific tissues—calcium and phosphorus are used to build teeth and bones. Others, such as iodine, are used to make hormones. Iron is one of the most important minerals for an athlete because it is a part of hemoglobin, which carries oxygen throughout the body (oxygen is needed by working muscles and all tissues). Minerals also regulate muscle contraction and body fluids, help transmit nerve impulses, and maintain a normal heart rhythm. Minerals are divided into two groups, macrominerals and trace minerals, depending on the body's needs (*Table 5.3*).

Table 5.3. Mineral Groups

Macrominerals (Body needs more)	*Trace Minerals (Body needs less)*
Calcium	Iron
Phosphorus	Manganese
Magnesium	Copper
Sodium	Iodine
Potassium	Zinc
Chloride	Cobalt
Sulfur	Fluoride
	Selenium

Eating too much of one mineral can interfere with the body's attempt to use another. For example, eating too much phosphorus can lower calcium levels and lead to bone loss; too much zinc can impair copper status. As with vitamins, eating more minerals does not speed up or improve how minerals work but instead can disturb the body's overall balance. *Tables 5.4* and *5.5* give food choices for three important minerals in the diets of young athletes—iron, zinc, and calcium.

The body's absorption of iron is influenced by many complex factors. Iron in meat is absorbed more easily than iron from plant sources. Foods that are rich in vitamin C (tomato, orange, melon, lemon, strawberries) help the body absorb iron.

Table 5.4. Iron and Zinc

Iron is important for healthy red blood cells (oxygen to muscles) and is found in:	*Zinc is important for healthy growth and development and is found in:*	*Both Iron and Zinc are found in:*
Enriched/whole-grain breads, pasta and cereals	Veal	Dry beans and peas
		Beef
	Bagels	Chicken
Beans (green, lima)	Bran muffin	Fish
Broccoli	Oat-ring cereals	Lamb
Spinach	Raisin bran	Pork
Potato with skin	Rice	Shellfish
Tomato juice		Turkey
Winter squash (acorn, butternut, etc)		Peas
Apricots (dried, canned)		Nuts
Prunes		
Raisins		

Nutrient Needs of Athletic Children

Athletic children do need some nutrients in higher amounts. They need extra calories and fluids to support their physical activity. Eating extra foods to provide enough energy usually supplies any additional vitamins or minerals that might be needed as well. However, years of scientific study have not demonstrated that athletic activity increases vitamin or mineral needs significantly. Feeding your young athletes a balanced diet of foods they like will give them enough of the vitamins and minerals that they need. There are lots of food alternatives for each vitamin and mineral. *Table 5.6* shows the wealth of vitamins and minerals that a healthful, balanced diet can supply even for the pickiest of eaters.

Table 5.5. Spotlight on Calcium

Children need at least three servings of calcium-rich foods each day so that:

- strong, hard bones grow
- teeth develop properly

Foods belonging to the Calcium Club include:

Milk	Cheese	Pudding
Custard	Yogurt	Ice cream
Milkshakes	Cheese pizza	Cream soups
Macaroni and cheese	Orange juice and fruit juice fortified with calcium	

Table 5.6. Vitamins and Minerals in Commonly Eaten Foods

Food	Vitamins and Minerals
Beef, chicken, fish, ham, pork, turkey	Iron, phosphorus, potassium, zinc, niacin, riboflavin, thiamin, vitamins B_6 and B_{12}
Peanut butter, almonds, walnuts, peanuts, seeds, other nuts	Copper, magnesium, phosphorus Vitamins A and B_{12}
Black beans, chick peas, kidney beans, lentils, navy beans, peas, pinto beans, soy beans	Iron, magnesium, phosphorus, potassium Folate
American, cottage, cheddar, part-skim mozzarella, ricotta, Swiss, and other cheese	Calcium, phosphorus Vitamins A and B_{12}
Bagels, corn bread, grits, crackers, pasta, corn muffins, noodles, pita bread, ready-to-eat cereal, white bread, rolls	Iron Thiamin, riboflavin, niacin
Brown rice, corn tortillas, oatmeal, whole-grain rye bread, whole-grain ready-to-eat cereal, whole-wheat pasta, crackers, bread, rolls	Copper, iron, magnesium, phosphorus, thiamin, riboflavin, niacin, vitamin E
Low-fat (1%) milk, low-fat flavored milk, skim milk, buttermilk, 2% milk, whole milk	Calcium, phosphorus, potassium, riboflavin; vitamins A, and D (if fortified)
Oranges, grapefruit, cantaloupe, watermelon, strawberries, blueberries, raspberries, tangerines	Potassium Folate, vitamins C and A (if deep yellow)
Apple, apricot, banana, cherries, fruit juice, grapes, peach, pear, pineapple, plum, prunes, raisins	Potassium Vitamins C and A (if deep yellow)
Broccoli, carrots, green pepper, kale, pumpkin, spinach, sweet potatoes, winter squash	Iron, magnesium, potassium Folate; riboflavin; vitamins A, C, K, E, and B_6
Black-eyed beans, corn, lima beans, green peas, potatoes	Iron, magnesium, phosphorus, potassium, folate
Cabbage, cauliflower, celery, cucumbers, green beans, lettuce, onions, summer squash, tomatoes, vegetable juice, zucchini	Magnesium, potassium Folate, vitamins C and K

Dietary Recommendations

Vitamin and mineral needs can be met easily by eating a well-balanced diet. Achieving such a diet over the long run is of major importance. Nutrient deficiencies develop over months, not days, and a healthy person can adapt to temporary shortages. More is not necessarily better! Young athletes can meet their vitamin and mineral needs on diets that include the foods and servings recommended in the Food Guide Pyramid.

Because children often do not eat enough fruits and vegetables in particular, they may be missing out on some important sources of vitamins and minerals. Review *Tables 5.7* and *5.8* to help children eat more fruits and vegetables.

Table 5.7. Eating Vegetables Can Be Fun!

Have children choose a vegetable at the grocery store and make it "veggie of the week."

Have children help plant and harvest a vegetable garden.

Let children help prepare vegetables for eating (washing, peeling, cooking).

Try dipping cut vegetables into yogurt, cheese, salsa, or bean dip.

Instead of serving the same vegetables prepared the same way, try new vegetables in new combinations and new cooking techniques:

- Stir-fry vegetables in a tablespoon of oil with small portions of meat or chicken.
- Add vegetables to chicken noodle soup.
- Lightly steam vegetables that you might normally serve raw.
- Replace carrot and celery sticks with raw cherry tomatoes, sugar-snap peas, green or red pepper strips, cauliflower or broccoli florets, summer squashes, radishes, or mushrooms.
- Add chopped green and red pepper to corn.
- Grate carrots and mix with raisins and apple chunks.
- Add chopped raw spinach and red cabbage to lettuce for a colorful salad.

Sprinkle grated cheese on top of steamed vegetables.

Offer vegetables at the beginning of a meal when children are hungriest and not filled up on other foods.

Serve small portions of vegetables cut in a variety of shapes.

Table 5.8. New Fruit Combos

Make frozen juice pops in an ice cube tray.

Freeze grapes, strawberries, bananas, and melon balls for frosty summer treats.

Try serving peaches or apricots with baked chicken or turkey, or add a pineapple slice to a hamburger!

continued

Table 5.8. New Fruit Combos... *(continued)*

Introduce children to unfamiliar fruits from other regions or nations, such as papaya, mango, kiwi, and figs.

Add fruit to gelatin molds.

Top pound cake or angel food cake with vanilla or lemon yogurt and fruit.

Select canned fruits packed in light syrup or natural juice rather than in heavy syrup.

Serve pineapple rings with a cherry in the middle.

Supplements Not Needed

Many well-meaning parents and coaches advise young athletes to take supplements as health insurance. Giving young athletes supplements can give them a false sense of security and may encourage future supplement use. They may assume that their morning dose of supplements provides them with all the vitamins and minerals they need so they can eat cookies and soda instead of fruit and yogurt.

Another disadvantage to using supplements is that athletes, particularly children, are likely to associate performance gains with whatever supplements they may happen to be taking. Of course, this is not true, but it may make children less willing to attribute gains to training, hard work, and a balanced diet. This type of false reinforcement also may make them try other types of supplements and substances (including, possibly, drugs and steroids), which can easily lead to a snowball effect with undesired consequences. Megadoses of supplements do not make up for lack of training or talent or give athletes a competitive edge.

To move away from this reliance on "supplement insurance," you must make your young athletes feel confident about eating "ordinary foods." If you continue to teach them how regular foods promote muscle growth and optimal performance, you can help them resist pressure to take supplements. You can do this by helping children keep records of what they eat, when and how hard they train, and how their athletic performance improves. Then you will be able to point to good dietary and training habits as the cause of any improvement, rather than leaving the children to associate good performance arbitrarily with a pill or powder. This approach empowers children to exert control over their athletic performance as well as in all areas of their lives.

Summary

Vitamins and minerals are substances that the body needs and can receive through a balanced diet. As with a car, overfilling the gas tank does not improve performance. In some cases, eating large amounts of certain vitamins and minerals can be dangerous. Young athletes should concentrate on eating a variety of foods to meet their vitamin and mineral needs.

Fluids

You might be surprised to learn that the most important part of any athlete's diet is fluids. While humans can survive for about a month without food, they can only survive a few days without water. Athletes need to drink extra fluids to replace body water lost while exercising. Child athletes must be especially careful to drink enough fluids while exercising. The type, amount, timing, and even the temperature of fluids consumed can affect how well the body rehydrates itself. As a coach or parent, you are responsible for preventing heat disorders in exercising children, and you must make sure that they drink enough fluids. This chapter addresses the special needs of younger athletes in maintaining proper body water levels.

Special Fluid Needs of Children

Compared with adults or even teenagers, preadolescent children need to be especially careful about drinking enough water for many reasons:

- Children do not tolerate temperature extremes well.
- Children sweat less.
- Children get hotter during exercise.
- Children have a lower cardiac output.
- Children have a greater relative surface area (more skin surface per body weight).

All these factors increase the risk of dehydration in children. Therefore, fluids play a critical role in maintaining the health and optimal performance of the child athlete. In addition, some sports require specific considerations regarding body water levels.

- Football and hockey players wear protective gear, which reduces the ability of the body to cool itself.

- Swimmers often do not realize that they are losing body water through sweat. They also can become dehydrated by sitting around in a hot, humid environment between sessions.

- Athletes in sports that have weight categories for competition (such as wrestling) *never* should deprive themselves of food or, especially, water to lose weight.

How Fluids Cool the Body

One of the most important functions of water is to cool the body. As a child exercises, heat generated by working muscles in turn raises the temperature of the entire body. When the body gets hot, it sweats, and as the sweat evaporates, the body is cooled. If the child does not replace this sweat by drinking more fluids, the body's water balance will be upset, and the body may soon overheat.

Humid days require even more care. If the air is humid, the sweat does not evaporate, and the body is not cooled. This can lead to overheating and heat disorders that may require medical attention.

How Much Water is Enough?

All athletes must drink water before, during, and after exercise. Dehydration can start when as little as 1% of body weight has been lost. In a 70-pound child, this would be less than 1 pound of weight loss. You should weigh young athletes before they train or compete and again during (if the session will be especially long) or after exercise so that you will know how much water they have lost. Follow the basic guidelines in *Table 6.1* to be sure that children are drinking enough water throughout an exercise session:

Give your young athletes personalized water bottles containing cold water and tell them to drink 3 to 4 ounces every 15 minutes.

Table 6.1. Guidelines for Drinking Water

Before Exercise	*During Exercise*	*After Exercise*
Drink 10–14 ounces of cold water 1–2 hours before the activity.	Drink 3–4 ounces of cold water every 15 minutes.	Drink 2 cups (16 ounces) of cold water for every pound of weight loss.
Drink 10 ounces of of cold water or diluted fruit juice 10-15 minutes before the activity		

You must watch and see how much water young athletes actually drink. Supervision is essential because children do not instinctively drink enough fluid to replace body water losses. Thirst does *not* indicate when an athlete needs to rehydrate; the body's thirst mechanism does not work well during exercise, and the athlete constantly must be reminded to drink. Children may not recognize the symptoms of heat strain and may push themselves to the point of heat injury.

Choosing the Right Fluids

Plain, cold water is the best and most economical source of fluid. Cold fluids are absorbed faster than warmer ones, and drinking water is the easiest way to rehydrate the body. Sports drinks (6% to 8% carbohydrate or 15 to 18 grams of carbohydrate per 1 cup),* which are made to encourage drinking fluids and replacing carbohydrate, also can be used, especially during activities lasting more than 90 minutes.

Even though water is adequate for most children, you will probably find that some are more likely to drink sufficient amounts if they are given flavored fluids. Sports drinks or diluted fruit juice are appropriate choices. Be sure to dilute fruit juice at least twofold: 1 cup of water for every 1 cup of juice. Tell children not to drink carbonated sodas or undiluted fruit juice as a fluid source during exercise. These beverages are too rich in carbohydrate (which can cause stomach cramps, nausea, and diarrhea), and caffeinated beverages (such as tea, coffee, and cola beverages) will dehydrate the body even more.

Foods that contain a lot of water, such as oranges, watermelon, apples, grapes, lettuce, and tomatoes, also can be used to rehydrate the body in conjunction with water. These foods provide water and carbohydrate and would be good choices to eat after exercising to replace lost water and lost energy (glycogen).

Salt Tablets

The recommendation here is simple: *Salt tablets should never be taken by athletes.*

Salt tablets contribute to dehydration because they cause extra water to enter the stomach and draw it away from other body tissues. They also irritate the stomach lining and can cause nausea.

You may have heard that muscle cramps are caused by inadequate salt intake, but they are more likely caused by large losses of water through excessive sweating. You should realize that sweat contains more water than sodium and potassium (electrolytes). The priority for any athlete should be to replace

*If products labeled "sports drinks" do not meet these guidelines, they may need to be diluted.

body water, not salt. Children will replace any electrolytes that they might have lost after exercise just by eating a healthful diet. Fruits and fruit juices are excellent sources of electrolytes.

Again, salt tablets never should be given to children. They *do not* help performance, but they *do* increase the risk for heat disorders and injury.

Dehydration and Heat Disorders

Dehydration is the loss of body fluid. If allowed to continue, this fluid loss not only affects athletic performance, it also becomes life-threatening. Exercising without drinking fluids dehydrates the body by itself. The body become dehydrated even faster under the following conditions:

- **Temperature**—The higher the temperature, the greater the sweat losses.

- **Humidity**—The higher the relative humidity, the greater the sweat losses.

- **Intensity**—The harder the athlete works, the greater the sweat losses. A *twofold* increase in speed produces a *fourfold* increase in sweat!

- **Body size**—The larger the athlete, the greater the sweat losses (boys generally sweat more than girls).

- **Duration**—The longer the workout, the greater the sweat losses.

- **Fitness**—Well-trained athletes sweat more, and they start sweating at a lower body temperature. Remember, the function of sweating is to cool the body, and the well-trained athlete cools his or her body more efficiently.

As water is lost during exercise, the body experiences a progression of heat-related illnesses. In addition to weighing young athletes before and after workouts and giving them personalized water bottles to drink from throughout exercise sessions, you must watch for the signs listed in *Table 6.2* and take appropriate action *immediately*.

Preventing Heat Disorders

In addition to making sure that your young athletes drink enough fluids, taking a number of precautions can reduce the risk of heat injury:

- Schedule workouts for the coolest times of the day (before 10 AM, after 6 PM), particularly in warmer climates. Take note of the humidity and air movement (wind) as well.

Table 6.2. Heat Disorders

Symptoms	Disorder	Treatment
Thirst Chills Clammy skin Throbbing heart Muscle pain, Spasms nausea	Heat cramps	Have the child drink 4–8 ounces of cold water every 10–15 minutes. Move the child to the shade and remove any excess clothing
Reduced sweating Dizziness Headache Shortness of breath Weak, rapid pulse Lack of saliva Extreme fatigue	Heat exhaustion	Stop exercise and move the child to a cool place. Have the child drink 16 ounces (2 cups) of water for every pound of weight lost. Take off the child's wet clothes and place an icebag on his or her head.
Lack of sweat Lack of urine Dry, hot skin Swollen tongue Visual disturbances (for example, seeing spots) Hallucinations Rapid pulse Unsteady gait Fainting Low blood pressure Loss of consciousness Shock	Heat stroke	Call for emergency medical treatment. Place ice bags on the back of the child's head. Remove the child's wet clothing. If the child is conscious, help him or her take a cold shower. If the child is in shock, elevate his or her feet. *Heat stroke ranks second among reported causes of death in high school athletes.*

◆ Allow children to adjust to warmer conditions gradually. Restrict the length and intensity of training sessions for the first 4 to 5 days and then increase the intensity slowly for another 1 to 2 weeks.

◆ Avoid excessive clothing, taping, or padding on hot or humid days. You can help improve body cooling by having the children change from sweaty clothes to dry ones. They should also wear white or light-colored clothing made of lightweight or mesh material and low-cut socks.

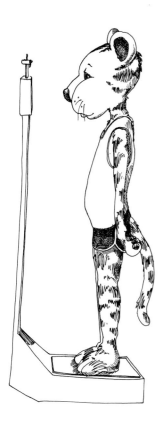

- Schedule breaks in the shade or other shelter. This will allow the children's bodies to cool down from the heat that built up during exercise.

- *Never* use water restrictions as a disciplinary measure. Water—preferably chilled water—*must* be available at all times during training and competition.

- Make sure that each child comes to practice or competition fully hydrated. Remind everyone in advance about how much water to drink before arriving.

- Weigh children before and throughout exercise to identify the ones who lose weight during practice or competition.

- Schedule water breaks during which all children must drink a minimum amount of water. Be especially strict with those who previously lost large amounts of weight during workouts.

- Pay close attention to children who are at risk for heat disorders due to obesity, poor conditioning, weight loss during exercise, or other health problems.

- Discourage the deliberate practice of dehydration. Tell young athletes that it keeps them from performing up to par athletically and can hurt their bodies seriously.

- Adjust the timing of practice and competition (time of day, season of year) as needed to prevent heat disorders. Extreme heat and/or humidity are valid reasons to cancel a scheduled workout or competition.

You should decide whether to modify or even cancel practice based on the air temperature and the humidity. You can do this most easily with a wet bulb thermometer (which measures both heat and humidity and is available at hardware stores). Specific guidelines for deciding whether to reduce exercise intensity or to cancel it altogether are as follows:

- If the wet bulb temperature is below 66°F, no precautions are necessary. Children who are susceptible to heat disorders should be watched closely.

- At a range of 66°F to 78°F, caution must be observed. Insist that unlimited amounts of water (preferably iced) be given, and monitor athletes closely for symptoms of heat disorders.

- Wet bulb temperatures above 78°F signify real danger for serious heat disorders. You must keep practice light, modifying or eliminating some routines as needed, and allow the athletes to work out in minimal gear. Water breaks in the shade are mandatory. Children who lose weight during exercise should be withdrawn from participation.

- The danger precautions just described also must be followed if the relative humidity is 95% or higher, regardless of the wet-bulb reading.

Summary

Coaches and trainers must supervise young athletes closely, making sure that they drink enough fluids to avoid dehydration. Weighing children before and after exercise is the best way to check whether they are drinking enough fluids to replace losses. In addition to adequate hydration before, during, and after exercise, young athletes must be educated on the danger associated with participating in extreme weight-loss practices that severely dehydrate the body.

CHAPTER 7

Pre- and Post-Event Meals

Before exercise, the time when child athletes eat is as important as *what* they eat. Of course, foods eaten routinely affect health and sports performance more than anything eaten the day of the event. As discussed in chapter 2, all athletes should eat most of their calories in the form of carbohydrate to store enough energy as glycogen. However, food eaten before, during, and after practice and competition can dramatically affect how an athlete feels while exercising. An upset stomach on game day usually results from poor food choices that morning. This chapter offers young athletes suggestions to plan appropriate pre- and post-event and training meals.

Pre-Event Meals

The pre-event meal serves two main purposes: first, to prevent athletes from feeling hungry before or during the event, and second, to help supply fuel to the muscles during training and competition. Still, most of the energy needed for any sports event is provided by whatever the athletes have eaten during the prior week. The best plan is to provide foods that children like and that contain lots of carbohydrate, low to moderate amounts of protein, and even less fat. Keep in mind the following guidelines:

♦ High-fat and high-protein foods take longer to digest than carbohydrate foods and, if eaten a few hours before exercising, can contribute to indigestion, nausea, and vomiting.

♦ To have a relatively empty stomach while exercising, the child should eat no sooner than 1 to 4 hours before practice or competition.

♦ Eating sugary foods such as candy and honey right before exercise does not provide quick energy.

Athletes should avoid eating simple carbohydrate (such as sugar, honey, candy, or soft drinks) for quick energy before exercise. Most of the energy for exercise comes from foods eaten several hours and days prior to the start of the event. Additionally, some athletes are more sensitive than others to changes in blood glucose levels when they eat simple sugars. Athletes should determine how sensitive they are to such changes by eating different amounts and sources of carbohydrate before exercising.

Table 7.1. Eating Before the Event

1-2 Hours Before	*2-3 Hours Before*	*3-4 Hours Before*
Fruit or vegetable juice	Fruit or vegetable juice	Fruit or vegetable juice
Fresh fruit (low fiber, eg, plums, melon, cherries, peaches)	Fresh fruit Breads, bagels, English muffins No margarine or cream cheese	Fresh fruit Breads, bagels, English muffins Peanut butter, lean meat, low-fat cheese Low-fat yogurt Baked potato Cereal with low-fat (1%) milk Pasta with tomato sauce

Sample Menus (3–4 Hours Before the Event)

1 cup orange juice Bagel 2 tablespoons peanut butter 2 tablespoons honey	1 cup orange juice $^3/_4$ cup corn flakes Medium banana Wheat toast and jelly 1 cup low-fat milk	1 cup orange juice Pancakes and syrup English muffin and jelly 1 cup low-fat yogurt	1 cup orange juice Waffles and strawberries 1 cup low-fat yogurt
1 cup vegetable soup 2 ounces skinless chicken 2 slices wheat bread 2 slices tomato 1 cup low-fat frozen yogurt 1 cup apple juice	Large baked potato 1 teaspoon margarine Carrot sticks $^1/_2$ cup fruit salad 1 cup low-fat milk	Salad: lettuce, 1 ounce ham, 1 ounce turkey, 2 slices tomato, carrot sticks, 2 tablespoons dressing $^1/_2$ cup pudding	2 cups spaghetti $^2/_3$ cup tomato sauce with mushrooms French bread 1 cup lemon sherbet 1 cup low-fat milk

Good sources of complex carbohydrate to eat before exercise include breads, pastas, rice, cereals, pancakes, rolls, bagels, English muffins, tortillas, fruits (bananas, apples, oranges), and vegetables (corn, peas, potatoes). These foods are all digested quickly, so that the athlete's stomach is empty and blood sugar level is stable by the time the practice or competition begins. Foods that are rich in carbohydrate also help to replenish energy (glycogen) stores, which may be required during prolonged training or competition. Read *Table 7.1* for suggestions on what to eat before exercising.

Sometimes children are too nervous or excited to eat on the day of an event. In this case, offer water and juice. Generally, however, you should be able to follow the simple pre-event guidelines in *Table 7.2*.

Table 7.2. Pre-Event Reminders

Eat	*Avoid*
Complex carbohydrate	Fat
Water	Protein
Moderate portions	Fiber
3–4 hours prior to event	Last-minute sweets

Eating at All-Day Events

During all-day events, whether competition or training, carbohydrate foods and drinks may delay the onset of fatigue. However, at regional tournaments, such as track, swimming, soccer, basketball, tennis, volleyball, or wrestling, nutritious food choices may be difficult to find, especially if the times at which events are held are likely to change. If possible, bring snacks for the team. Otherwise, children need to make wise choices at concession stands or bring snacks from home.

The "Instead of" foods listed in *Table 7.3* will stay in the stomach longer and impair performance. School-aged athletes do not need electrolytes; therefore, sports drinks are not necessary, but the flavor may encourage children to drink more fluids. Just be sure that the carbohydrate level is not too concentrated (no more than 6% to 8%, or 15 to 18 grams of carbohydrate per cup).

Table 7.3. If You're Going To Compete

Try . . .	*Instead of . . .*
Bagels	Candy bars
Bananas	Doughnuts
Fruit juice	French fries
Muffins	Hot dogs
Pretzels (hard or soft)	Nachos
Sports drinks	Potato chips
(6%–8% carbohydrate)	Soda

Post-Event Meals

As soon as children stop exercising, give them water and fruit juices for rehydration and complex carbohydrate sources to replenish glycogen stores. The body is most efficient at absorbing and storing energy (glycogen) during the first 4 to 5 hours after exercise. In fact, the post-event meal is probably more important than the pre-event meal because it determines how much energy an athlete will have for the next training session or competition. Foods and fluids to be eaten immediately after training or competing include the following:

- Medium bagel (50 grams carbohydrate)
- Pretzels (23 grams carbohydrate per 1 ounce)
- Fruit yogurt (40 grams carbohydrate per 8 ounces)
- Large banana (40 grams carbohydrate)
- Cranberry-apple juice (43 grams carbohydrate per 8 ounces)
- Apple juice (30 grams carbohydrate per 8 ounces)
- Orange juice (28 grams carbohydrate per 8 ounces)

About 2 hours after exercising, child athletes should eat a meal that contains mostly carbohydrate: yogurt and fruit, cheese and bagel, vegetable pizza, or spaghetti and meat sauce. You can follow the guidelines given for pre-event meals and include more protein and fat.

Summary

What and when an athlete eats on game day is important, and child athletes should be taught early the healthful and scientific way to improve performance through diet, rather than be allowed to develop superstitious and potentially harmful routines on their own. As with the daily diet, carbohydrate (especially complex carbohydrate) foods should be emphasized prior to and after training and competing. It may seem that a quick snack just before lining up should give athletes an extra boost, but it may, in fact, slow them down. The post-event meal is important for restoring energy to athletes' muscles. The basic rules for eating before and after exercise are simple, easy to follow, and not mysterious or magical in the least.

CHAPTER

8

Meals on the Go

We Americans are eating more and more of our meals on the go. A 1990 Gallup survey indicated that Americans eat out an average of 3.7 times per week. Until recently, there were few nutritious, balanced food choices available in fast-food restaurants. In the past few years, however, fast-food franchises and family-style restaurants began to take healthful eating seriously and added more low-fat foods to their menus. Now, convenience foods can be nutritious and fit in any budget. This chapter offers simple guidelines for making healthful food choices away from home.

Fast Food

Many coaches and parents choose convenience foods for child athletes because of tight time schedules. Although the amount of time available may seem to outweigh nutrition considerations, they need not conflict. Fast-food establishments provide quick service, inexpensive meals, and consistent food quality at easily accessible locations. Although many fast foods still have too much fat and salt and not enough vitamins, minerals, and fiber, many franchises now offer low-fat, nutritious food choices as well.

When stopping at a fast-food restaurant, remember to focus on finding carbohydrate foods. As a coach or parent, you can help children order low-fat, high-carbohydrate items. Be sure to be a role model yourself! The handout on individual food items and toppings should be helpful. In addition, *Table 8.1* lists meal plans to encourage and to discourage.

Table 8.1. Fast-Food Meal Plans

Go for It!	*Stop and Think Again!*
Pancakes with syrup Low-fat (1%) milk Orange juice	Biscuit with egg, cheese, and bacon Whole milk
Baked potato with chili Roll with 1 pat margarine Garden salad, 1/4 packet dressing Low-fat yogurt milkshake	Deluxe double cheeseburger Large French fries Regular soda Apple pie or turnover
Thick-crust vegetable pizza Bread sticks Garden salad, 1 ladle dressing Low-fat (1%) milk	Double cheese, double pepperoni pizza Fried mozzarella cheese Regular soda
Single hamburger Muffin Orange juice	Hot dog with chili and cheese Onion rings Chocolate malt

Family-Style Restaurants

Family-style restaurants offer a wider variety of nutritionally sound choices. Eating a meal together before or after a game or competition can be an enjoyable experience for children, parents, and coaches. Once again, remember that children learn good dining habits by watching adults select healthful food items.

Breakfast items, such as pancakes, cereal, bagels, and English muffins, are an inexpensive and easy way to select high-carbohydrate meals. Many other menu items that children enjoy will also offer sound sports nutrition. Consider the lunch or dinner menus listed in *Table 8.2* and why they would or would not be good for athletes in training.

Table 8.2. Family-Style Restaurant Meal Plans

Go for It!	*Stop and Think Again!*
Roast beef sandwich (lettuce and tomato) Fruit juice Low-fat vanilla milkshake	Fried fish with tartar sauce Onion rings Soda
Spaghetti with tomato sauce Bread with 1 pat margarine Garden salad, 1 ladle dressing Fruit cup Low-fat (1%) milk	Crispy fried chicken Mashed potatoes with butter and gravy Biscuits with butter Whole milk

Grocery and Convenience Stores

Where can you buy food for the young athlete at an all-day soccer tournament? Grocery stores, convenience stores, and concession stands are usually the choices available; unfortunately, they typically offer high-fat, non-nutritious foods. Well, maybe not. Grocery and convenience stores often are overlooked as a source of quick, inexpensive, nutritious snacks and meals. With guidance from coaches and parents, young athletes can choose from among fruits, juices, muffins, and low-fat dairy products rather than candy bars, snack chips, and soft drinks. Make looking for snacks fun! In addition to finding something good to drink (low-fat milk, juice, water), ask the child to find a food that is creamy, crunchy, and juicy *(Table 8.3)*.

Table 8.3. Grocery Store Snack Suggestions

Creamy	*Crunchy*	*Juicy*
Low-fat cheese	Carrots	Oranges
Yogurt	Apple	Peaches
Banana	Crackers	Plums
Peanut butter	Pretzels	Watermelon
	Cereal	Berries
	Popcorn	

Sometimes special requests to the event organizers for specific food items, for example, fruit juice, fruit, and bread products) will be honored. If the host of the tournament or race does not plan to offer nutritionally sound foods, be sure to bring a cooler of high-performance snacks or to locate a nearby source of low-fat, high-carbohydrate foods.

Summary

Providing all young athletes with food guidelines will help them to pick out high-performance foods from almost any menu or food aisle. Diets that are high in carbohydrate and fluids, moderate in protein, and low in fat will give child athletes enough calories and nutrients to grow, train, and compete. Finding such high-performance choices at fast-food establishments, family-style restaurants, and grocery stores takes practice but can be done. Usually you can request brochures that provide nutrition information from fast-food franchises. If the restaurant manager does not have any in the store, he or she can give you the address to write to for more information.

Of course, it is also important to let kids be kids (see Table 1). An occasional ice cream cone, candy bar, or bag of chips is completely acceptable. However, they should be eaten occasionally *in addition* to high-performance foods, not *in place* of them!

Body Weight and the Child Athlete

Is there really an "ideal" body weight for competition? The athlete, coach, or parent who thinks so may believe that reaching a certain body weight will make a child more competitive. Attaining a "competitive" weight might mean gaining or losing weight for an imagined competitive edge. However, as the child progresses in a sport, he or she may develop compulsive eating behaviors and become obsessed with reaching and maintaining a specific "competitive" weight. Add the irregular eating schedules, meal skipping, and excessive snacking common among all children, and the potential for problems begins to snowball.

More than ever, children are experimenting with fad diets, diet pills, and weight-gain powders and pills, all of which are dangerous in growing bodies. Such extreme eating behaviors also can lead to eating disorders, such as anorexia nervosa and bulimia nervosa. Determining whether a child needs to gain or lose weight and then deciding how to do it is quite a challenge and should not be undertaken without supervision by a pediatrician and a registered dietitian. This chapter addresses the issues of attaining a "competitive" weight and reviews appropriate methods for gaining or losing weight. It also lists the early signs, symptoms, and approaches for dealing with disordered eating behaviors.

Losing Fat

You have probably seen it happen. As competition day approaches, a young athlete may panic, feeling that he or she is too fat to win. In some cases it may be true, but the days and even weeks prior to competition are the worst times to start trying to lose weight. A starved athlete may not perform effectively, and one who has attempted an unsafe weight-loss method will be even more disadvantaged. As discussed in chapter 1, young children need a certain amount of food calories that provide energy to grow normally.

You must be aware that some young athletes may experiment with diuretics, starvation or fad diets, or other methods to lose weight quickly. Rapid weight loss usually rids the body of water weight and possibly even lean body tissue from muscles or vital organs. For any athlete, these methods lead to dehydration, low muscle glycogen stores, fatigue, and poor performance. For the still-growing child athlete, the risks are even greater. *Table 9.1* lists some tips for working with an overweight child.

Table 9.1. Working With an Overweight Child

Parents	*Coaches*
Consult with a registered dietitian if you think your child might have a weight problem.	Do not single out the overweight child by making him or her run extra laps or exercise longer.
Do not single out the overweight child in the family by serving special foods or imposing restrictions.	Never restrict fluids for any child.
	Never refer to a child as overweight, especially in front of his or her teammates.
Encourage the overweight child to eat slowly and to enjoy whatever he or she eats.	Watch for signs of heat distress. Overweight children are at higher risk for heat disorders than thinner children.
Never give food as a reward or withhold it as a punishment.	Be patient!
Be a role model: exercise and eat a balanced, low-fat diet yourself.	Be a role model: eat a balanced diet, keep active, and maintain a healthy body weight.
Do not tell a child that he or she is "on a diet."	

Many children will attain their goal weights simply by making changes in their diets and exercising more. Replacing high-calorie, high-fat foods with nutritious, low-calorie, high-carbohydrate foods improves athletic performance, produces some weight loss, and helps steer them toward a healthy life-style so they can gradually "grow into" their weight. However, when weight loss or fat loss is considered necessary by the pediatrician and registered dietitian, diet alone is not an effective method for reducing body fat. Exercise is also important. The following guidelines will help young athletes lose weight gradually and safely:

Setting goals

♦ Because each child is unique, there is no such thing as an "ideal" body weight. Young athletes should strive to achieve a weight that feels good and gives them the energy and stamina that they need to train and compete.

- Only health-care experts, such as pediatricians and registered dietitians, should recommend a specific goal body weight. They can take into consideration the child's level of sexual maturation, growth, and development. Many times the child athlete may not need to lose weight but instead needs to grow to a height that is appropriate for his or her weight.

- Weight loss goals must be realistic and achievable—usually not more than 10% of body weight at a time. Otherwise, a child could become frustrated, particularly if he or she has trouble keeping the weight off later.

- Goal weight should be achieved at least 3 to 4 weeks prior to the start of training and competition. This will help children participate at peak performance.

Less energy in (eat less) + more energy out (exercise more) → fat loss

- Cut back on foods that provide empty calories (for example, sodas, candy bars, chips, cookies, and emphasize low-fat foods from the food groups featured in the Food Guide Pyramid.

- Weight loss should be slow—no more than $\frac{1}{2}$ to 1 pound per week.

- Exercise more often for longer periods, but only at moderate intensity (heart rate of about 130 beats per minute).

- Do aerobic exercise, such as fast walking, running, hiking, biking, swimming, or other continuous rigorous activity.

- Choose family activities that include exercise. Excessive television watching—even if the entire family is present—can affect children's eating habits *(Table 9.2)*.

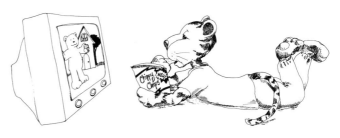

Table 9.2. Television and Weight Control

For the entire family, discourage eating meals or snacks while watching television.

Watch television with children. Discuss advertisements and how they can be misleading.

Be selective about what children watch on television and limit the time they spend in front of the television or playing video games.

Specific strategies

- ◆ Eat three servings of low-fat milk products (1 serving = 8 ounces of milk or yogurt, or 1½ to 2 ounces cheese).

- ◆ Eat two to three servings of lean meats, poultry, or fish (1 serving = 2 to 3 ounces cooked lean meat).

- ◆ Eat two to four or more servings of fruits (1 serving = 1 medium fruit, ½ cup chopped, or ¾ cup juice).

- ◆ Eat three to five servings of vegetables (not fried, no added sauces, no butter or margarine; 1 serving = ½ cup cooked or raw, ¾ cup of juice).

- ◆ Eat six to eleven servings of breads, cereals, pasta, rice, or other grains (skip pastries; 1 serving = 1 slice of bread, ½ cup cooked cereal, rice or pasta, or 1 ounce of ready-to-eat cereal).

- ◆ Eat at regular intervals—three meals plus planned snacks—to avoid hunger and impulse eating. *Table 9.3* presents a sample menu for one day.

- ◆ Stick to a planned exercise schedule that includes at least **three** aerobic workouts per week that last more than 30 minutes.

Table 9.3. Sample Menu for Weight Control

Breakfast

¾ cup orange juice
¾ cup raisin bran (1 teaspoon sugar optional)
1 slice whole-wheat toast
1 tablespoon jam or jelly
1 cup low-fat (1%) milk

Lunch

1 turkey sandwich
   3 ounces turkey breast
   2 slices whole-wheat bread
   mustard
   sliced tomato and lettuce
1 apple
1 cup low-fat (1%) milk

Snack

1 banana

Dinner

3 ounces lean beef
1 medium baked potato
½ cup plain non-fat yogurt
½ cup green beans
1 cup low-fat (1%) milk
½ cup ice milk

Snack

¾ cup tomato juice
1 ounce pretzels
¼ cup raisins

Gaining Weight

Gaining weight can give too-thin child athletes the competitive edge to win. To gain weight, the children must consume more calories than they use for growth and in exercise, and also must continue to exercise to prevent gaining weight as fat, rather than as muscle. Of course, as discussed in chapter 1, only children who have reached puberty have the hormones to build larger, stronger muscles. For example, boys who are too young to add muscle mass should not be fed more protein foods in an attempt to "bulk them up" for sports like football or hockey.

Extra calories should come mainly from additional carbohydrate. Protein levels should remain at recommended dietary intakes for the athlete's age and gender, and fat intake should be adjusted only to continue providing 30% of calories as fat. The following guidelines will help young athletes gain weight appropriately:

Setting goals

♦ Goals must be realistic, particularly because children already require a lot of food, and eating even more to gain weight may be difficult.

♦ Only health-care experts, such as pediatricians and registered dietitians, should recommend a specific goal body weight. They can take into consideration the child's level of sexual maturation, growth, and development.

♦ Gaining weight slowly and steadily means adding less body fat and more lean body weight, or muscle. No more than 1/2 to 1 pound should be gained each week.

More food in (change in diet) + muscle use (exercise) ➔ lean body weight gain

♦ Children who train at a competitive level may need to eat as many as 3000 to 5000 Calories every day to gain weight.

♦ Children should increase portion sizes and eat more snacks between meals to gain weight; alternatively, they can eat smaller amounts more often (five to six feedings) throughout the day.

♦ Children who eat to gain weight should take care not to eat too much fat (particularly saturated fat) and cholesterol.

♦ In adolescents, weight-training exercises that work muscles to fatigue add bulk and strength while increasing body weight.

Specific strategies

◆ Eat a large bedtime snack that includes food from all food groups (for example, a peanut butter and banana sandwich with low-fat milk).

◆ Eat foods with plenty of complex and simple carbohydrates (for example, pancakes and syrup, orange juice, low-fat milk, pizza, and low-fat milkshakes). A sample day's menu is given in *Table 9.4.*

◆ Use weight-gain supplements only if recommended by a pediatrician or registered dietitian. *Drinks* are expensive, but it is sometimes easier to drink 500 Calories than to eat them. One suggestion is a powdered breakfast mix made with low-fat milk. *Snack bars* are also expensive and usually provide no more calories than a store-bought breakfast or granola bar eaten with a glass of low-fat milk. *Powders* are very expensive and usually are made just of egg white solids, soy protein or dry milk, and a carbohydrate source.

Table 9.4. Sample Menu for Weight Gain

Breakfast
1 cup orange juice
6 pancakes
$^1/_4$ cup syrup
2 pats margarine
$1^1/_2$ cup low-fat (1%) milk

Snack
1 soft pretzel
$1^1/_2$ cup tomato juice

Lunch
1 turkey sandwich
    4–5 ounces turkey breast
    1 7-in pita bread pocket
    2 tablespoons light mayonnaise
    chopped tomato and lettuce
1 cup fruit yogurt
2 cups apple juice
1 large muffin

Snack
1 package powdered breakfast mix
1 cup low-fat (1%) milk

Dinner
1 medium vegetable-cheese pizza
2 cups low-fat (1%) milk

Snack
1 peanut butter and jelly sandwich
    3 tablespoons peanut butter
    3 tablespoons jelly
    2 slices whole-grain bread
1 cup low-fat (1%) milk

Eating Disorders Among Athletes

Some athletes try to become thin at any cost. Often one of those costs is the development of an eating disorder. Disordered eating behaviors may be triggered by many factors:

♦ crash dieting;
♦ intense desire for athletic success;
♦ fear of failure;
♦ a seemingly harmless comment by a coach or parent about the athlete's weight; and
♦ frustration or guilt about not being able to control body weight.

Because inappropriate dieting rituals often are continued into adulthood, you must teach young athletes early in their careers about the dangers of eating disorders and about healthy methods for controlling their body weight. Look over the lists of warning signs for two major eating disorders—anorexia nervosa and bulimia nervosa—so that you can recognize potential problems in your young athletes *(Table 9.5).* Note, however, that the presence of just one or two of these symptoms does not necessarily indicate the presence of an eating disorder. Children should always be seen by appropriate health professionals—a pediatrician, registered dietitian, or psychologist—before a diagnosis is made.

Table 9.5. Eating Disorders

Anorexia Nervosa	*Bulimia Nervosa*
Sudden, large weight loss	Noticeable weight loss or gain
Preoccupation with food, calories, and weight	Excessive concern about weight
Wears baggy or layered clothing	Visits bathrooms after meals
	Depressive moods
Relentless, excessive exercise	Strict dieting followed by eating binge
Mood swings	Increasingly criticizes his or her body
Avoids food-related social activities	

Coaching Your Athlete

As a coach or parent, you can dramatically influence the eating and exercise behaviors of young athletes. Be careful about what you say, especially about body size. Strong athletes are better than scrawny athletes, but children should not start trying to bulk up before they are the right age, either. The following pointers may help you understand or identify athletes at risk for eating disorders:

♦ The better you know your athletes, the more help you will be to them. Watch for any physical or, possibly, emotional changes that your athletes may display.

- Discuss nutrition issues, eating habits, and weight concerns openly. Encourage athletes to come to you with any questions they might have or to ask advice.

- If you think any of your athletes has an eating disorder or a distorted body image (believing they are fatter than they really are), let them know that they can come to you privately and that they can trust you to keep what they say confidential. They often want help but do not know how to ask.

- If you identify a problem or feel unable to help, encourage the athlete to talk to his or her pediatrician. Early identification and treatment are key to helping any athlete with an eating disorder.

The following pointers may help you prevent eating disorders:

- Adults should be role models for healthy attitudes toward eating and body image.

- Encourage children to eat according to their appetites. Never withhold food or force children to eat.

- Teach children to feel good about themselves, regardless of body size or shape.

Food should *never* be used as a punishment or reward.

Summary

Young athletes who receive nutrition and fitness education are less likely to develop eating disorders or body weight problems. Once they recognize that a certain percentage of body fat is healthy and even required for optimal performance, child athletes are better able to resist the temptation of becoming thin at all costs. A "competitive" weight can be achieved through a sound, balanced diet and an appropriate training program. Whether trying to lose or gain weight, children need support and guidance from their parents, coaches, and health-care professionals.

◆◆

Answers to Handout Puzzles

Carbohydrate: The Energy Booster

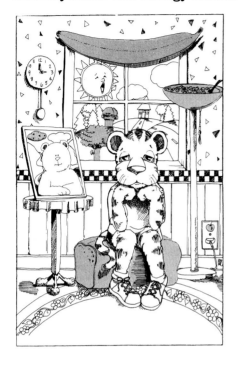

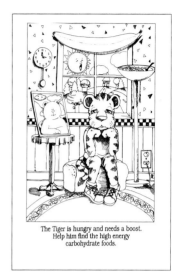

The Tiger is hungry and needs a boost. Help him find the high energy carbohydrate foods.

Protein: The Body's Building Block

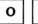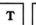

P R O T E I N

B U I L D I N G

B L O C K S

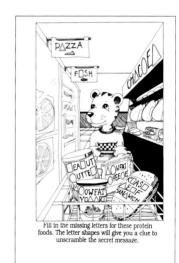

Fill in the missing letters for these protein foods. The letter shapes will give you a clue to unscramble the secret message.

Attack the Fat

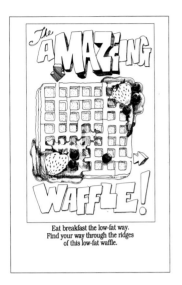

Eat breakfast the low-fat way.
Find your way through the ridges
of this low-fat waffle.

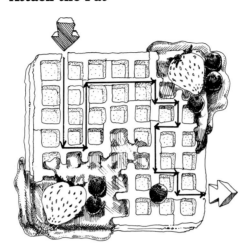

Vitamins and Minerals

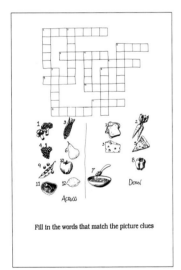

Fill in the words that match the picture clues

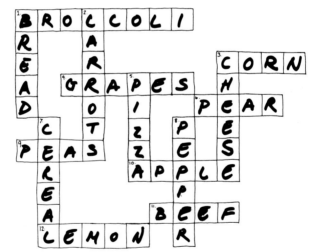

Fluids

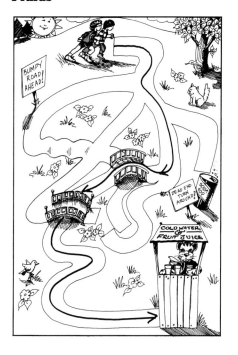

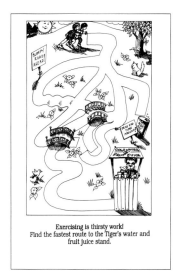

Exercising is thirsty work!
Find the fastest route to the Tiger's water and
fruit juice stand.

Good Food Fast

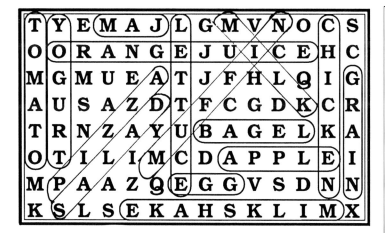

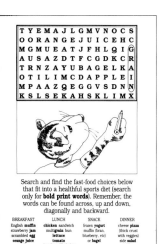

```
T Y E M A J L G M V N O C S
O O R A N G E J U I C E H C
M G M U E A T J F H L Q I G
A U S A Z D T F C G D K C R
T R N Z A Y U B A G E L K A
O T I L I M C D A P P L E I
M P A A Z Q E G G V S D N N
K S L S E K A H S K L I M X
```

Search and find the fast-food choices below
that fit into a healthful sports diet (search
only for **bold print words**). Remember, the
words can be found across, up and down,
diagonally and backward.

BREAKFAST	LUNCH	SNACK	DINNER
English **muffin**	**chicken** sandwich	frozen **yogurt**	cheese **pizza**
strawberry **jam**	multi**grain** bun	muffin (bran,	(thick crust
scrambled **egg**	**lettuce**	blueberry, etc)	with veggies)
orange juice	**tomato**	or **bagel**	side **salad**
milk	low-fat **milkshake**		**milk**
	apple brought from home		

The Weight Balance

<u>E</u>   <u>A</u>   T   <u>R</u>   <u>I</u>   <u>G</u>   <u>H</u>   T   <u>&</u>

<u>E</u>   <u>X</u>   <u>E</u>   <u>R</u>   <u>C</u>   <u>I</u>   <u>S</u>   <u>E</u>

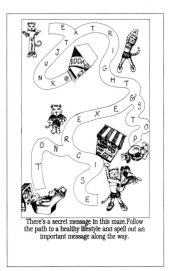

There's a secret message in this maze. Follow the path to a healthy lifestyle and spell out an important message along the way.

◆◆◆

Reproducible Masters for Handouts

Carbohydrate: The Energy Booster (chapter 2)

Protein: The Body's Building Block (chapter 3)

Attack the Fat (chapter 4)

Vitamins and Minerals (chapter 5)

Fluids (chapter 6)

Eat to Compete (chapter 7)

Good Food Fast (chapter 8)

The Weight Balance (chapter 9)

CARBOHYDRATE: The Energy Booster

 • Is there one BEST food for my child to eat in order to • boost performance?

Instead of only one food, there is one best TYPE of food; CARBO-HYDRATE. These foods are best because they are the preferred fuel for exercise. By feeding your child fruits and vegetables, low-fat milk and other dairy foods, and breads and cereals; you can be sure your child's diet contains adequate carbohydrates for performance.

 •My child's favorite carbohydrate foods are ice cream and • candy. Does it matter whether the carbohydrates are "simple" or "complex"?

Simple carbohydrates or simple sugars often taste sweet. They are easily digested and absorbed into the bloodstream to provide quick energy. Examples are milk, fruit and "sweets" like candy and cookies.

Complex carbohydrates are starchy foods. They provide energy more slowly because they take longer to be digested. They carry other nutrients like fiber, vitamins, and minerals along with them. Because they carry these other nutrients, they would be more healthful and should be eaten most of the time.

 • I've always heard that carbohydrate foods like bread and • potatoes are fattening. What is the real story?

Bread and potatoes are both excellent sources of carbohydrate. "Fattening" would only apply to these carbohydrates if they were eaten in excess quantity or with high-fat toppings such as margarine, sour cream, or bacon. If the excess energy was not required for the child's growth and activity, it would be stored as fat in the child's body.

SAMPLE MENU LOADED WITH CARBOHYDRATE

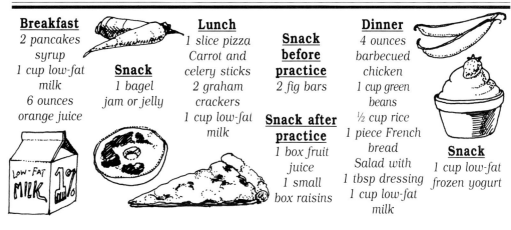

Breakfast
2 pancakes
syrup
1 cup low-fat
milk
6 ounces
orange juice

Snack
1 bagel
jam or jelly

Lunch
1 slice pizza
Carrot and
celery sticks
2 graham
crackers
1 cup low-fat
milk

Snack before practice
2 fig bars

Snack after practice
1 box fruit
juice
1 small
box raisins

Dinner
4 ounces
barbecued
chicken
1 cup green
beans
½ cup rice
1 piece French
bread
Salad with
1 tbsp dressing
1 cup low-fat
milk

Snack
1 cup low-fat
frozen yogurt

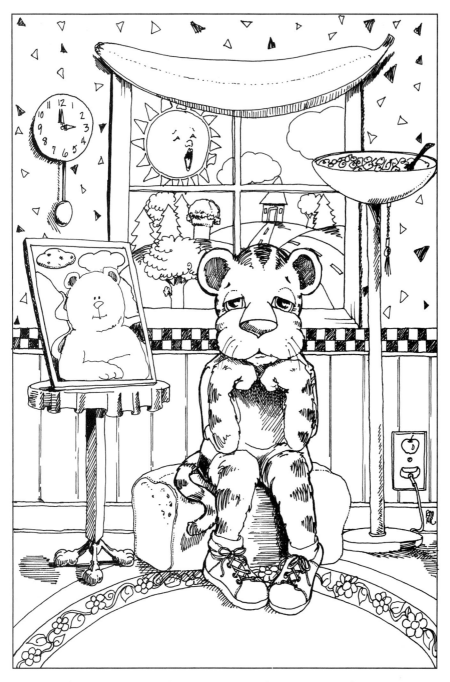

The Tiger is hungry and needs a boost.
Help him find the high energy
carbohydrate foods.

loaf of bread, bowl of cereal, apple, banana,
broccoli, potato, ice cream cone

PROTEIN: The Body's Building Block

 • How do the protein building blocks work together?

Protein building blocks come from the foods we eat. They work together to build and maintain the body. In other words . . .

Protein:
- ✦ maintains and repairs muscle.
- ✦ makes hemoglobin which gets oxygen to the body.
- ✦ forms antibodies in the blood that fight off infection and disease.
- ✦ produces enzymes and hormones that regulate body processes.
- ✦ can supply energy when necessary.

 • But I thought protein causes muscle growth, too. If protein doesn't, what does?

Protein does provide the building blocks for muscular growth, but muscular growth comes from . . .

BASIC DIET + LEVEL OF MATURATION* + TRAINING + TRAINING =
MUSCULAR GROWTH

*Level of maturation: This depends on whether the athlete has reached the stage of maturation in which the hormones are released in sufficient amounts to add muscle mass.

 • How do I make sure my child gets enough dietary protein?

The Dietary Guidelines for Americans suggest that children between the ages of 6 to 12 years get FOUR (8-ounce) servings of milk daily and TWO to THREE daily servings of other protein foods such as meat, eggs, dry beans, and nuts. If the child athlete regularly consumes this, his or her protein needs will be met.

HIGH PROTEIN AFTER SCHOOL MUNCHIES

CRUNCHY PEANUT BUTTER SANDWICH

2 slices hearty, whole-grain bread
2 tbsp crunchy peanut butter
2 tbsp low-fat granola
½ banana, sliced

1. Spread peanut butter on the bread.
2. Sprinkle the granola on top of the peanut butter.
3. You may add sliced banana to soothe the sweet tooth.

Nutrition Info: Calories: 473 protein: 17.2 g (14%)
      carbohydrate: 62.8 g (49%) fat: 20.8 g (37%)

FRUITY FIZZ

1 cup low-fat vanilla yogurt
½ cup berries;
      (strawberries, blueberries, etc)
½ cup seltzer

1. Combine yogurt and fruit in blender; blend well.
2. Add seltzer; blend again 2–3 seconds to fizz.

Nutrition Info: Calories: 227 protein: 11.9 g (20%)
      carbohydrate: 39.3 g (67%) fat :3.3 g (13%)

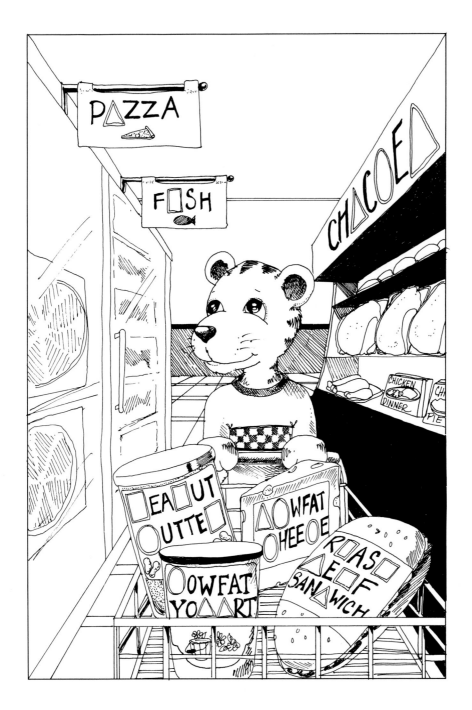

Fill in the missing letters for these protein foods. The letter shapes will give you a clue to unscramble the secret message.

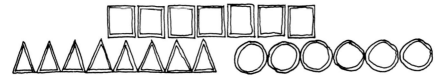

ATTACK THE FAT

 • What is FAT?

Fat is a source of stored energy found in the muscle and under the skin. Fat is also found in many of the foods we eat—animal and plant foods. Each gram of dietary fat yields 9 Calories. The majority of an athlete's dietary fat should be of the heart-healthy varieties; mono-unsaturated and polyunsaturated fats.

 • Is it true that kids need a certain amount of fat to grow?

Yes. Kids do need dietary fat to grow appropriately. Fats are a source of essential fatty acids necessary for growth. Dietary fats also aid in the absorption of the fat-soluble vitamins A, D, E, and K. The American Academy of Pediatrics recommends that growing kids get 30% of their daily calories from dietary fats.

 • Can I trust food labels to give me guidance on low-fat • foods?

In the past, many food labels did not tell the whole story. With the NEW food labels of 1993, much of the confusion has been removed. Food labels can help you make healthy food choices for your family. Children often make high-fat food choices with convienience foods, but by reading food labels and becoming aware of serving sizes and fat content you can balance your child's plate. An occasional high-fat but nutritious food such as pizza can be balanced with a low-fat salad to help your child have a healthful diet.

FIGHT FAT . . . THINK AGAIN

BREAKFAST		LUNCH/ DINNER	
Instead of . . .	*Try . . .*	*Instead of . . .*	*Try . . .*
Sausage biscuit	Waffle with fruit	Fried chicken	Grilled chicken
Hash browns	Grits or oatmeal	sandwich	sandwich without
Whole milk	Orange juice		mayo sauce
	Low-fat milk	French fries	Pretzels
		Chocolate cake	Apple
		Regular milkshake	Low-fat yogurt shake

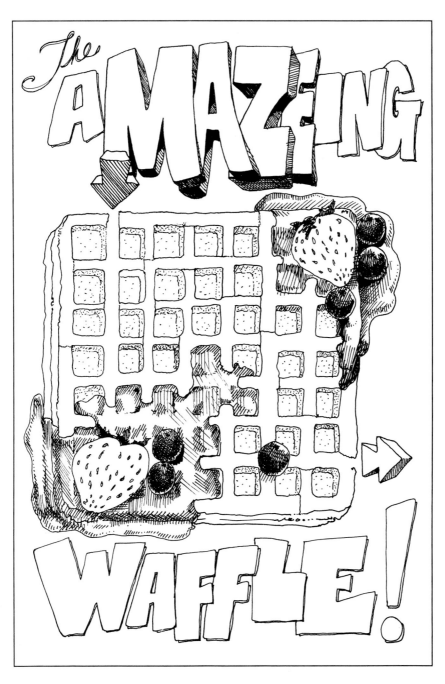

Find your way through the ridges
of this low-fat waffle and eat breakfast the
low-fat way. With delicious toppings such as
strawberries and blueberries, who needs to
eat the high-fat way?

VITAMINS AND MINERALS

 : Vitamins and minerals; are they magic or metabolic?

Vitamins and minerals are complex organic substances found in tiny quantities in the foods we eat. They do not contain energy but they do work together in the body to help maintain health and promote growth and development of children. So, they are not magic, but yes, they are metabolic and help the body function properly.

 : If a little is good, will more be better?

Other than deficiency diseases, vitamins and minerals have not been shown to prevent or cure any disease, including the common cold. Supplementation will not cause the child to mature faster or become stronger. Encouraging supplementation is also teaching the child athlete to rely on a supplement as "insurance" of an athletic success rather than attributing the success to training, hard work and a balanced diet.

 : My child won't eat vegetables. Should I give a supplement to replace these nutrients?

Vitamin and mineral supplements should NOT be used to replace food or make up for poor dietary habits. The following table shows the great variety of food choices that supply the vitamins and minerals your child athlete needs.

Apple, apricot, banana, cherries, fruit juice, grapes, peach, pear, pineapple, plum, prunes, raisins Potassium, vitamin C, (if deep yellow) A	*Oranges, grapefruit, cantaloupe, watermelon, strawberries, blueberries, raspberries, tangerines* Potassium, folate, vitamin C, (if deep yellow) A	*Black beans, chickpeas, kidney beans, lentils, navy beans, peas, pinto beans, soy beans* Iron, magnesium, phosphorus, potassium, folate
Broccoli, carrots, green pepper, kale, pumpkin, spinach, sweet potatoes, winter squash Iron, magnesium, phosphorus, potassium, folate, vitamins A and C	*Brown rice, oatmeal, corn tortillas, whole-grain breads, whole-grain cereals, whole-wheat pastas and crackers* Copper, iron, magnesium, phosphorus, thiamin, riboflavin, niacin, vitamin E	*American, cottage, cheddar, part-skim mozzarella, ricotta, Swiss, and other cheeses* Calcium, phosphorus, vitamins A and B$_{12}$
Black-eyed peas, corn, lima beans, green peas, potatoes Iron, magnesium, phosphorus, potassium, folate		*Bagels, cornbread, grits, crackers, pasta, noodles, pita bread, ready-to-eat cereals, white bread, rolls* Iron, thiamin, riboflavin, niacin
Cabbage, cauliflower, celery, cucumbers, green beans, lettuce, onions, summer squash, tomatoes, vegetable juice, zucchini Magnesium, potassium, folate, vitamins C and K	*Beef, chicken, pork, turkey, ham* Iron, phosphorus, potassium, zinc, niacin, riboflavin, thiamin, vitamins B$_6$ and B$_{12}$	*Low-fat milk, low-fat flavored milk, skim milk, buttermilk, whole milk* Calcium, phosphorus, potassium, riboflavin, vitamins B$_{12}$, A, and (if fortified) D
	Peanut butter, seeds, almonds, walnuts, peanuts, other nuts Copper, magnesium, phosphorus, vitamins A and B$_{12}$	

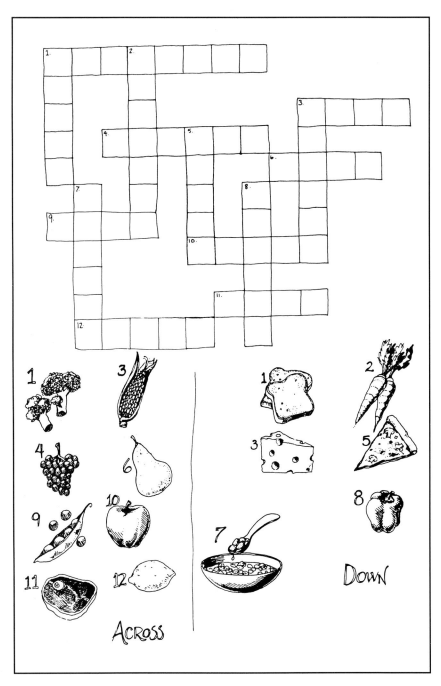

These foods are loaded with vitamins and minerals. Fill in the words that match the picture clues then find these foods in the table on the other side and learn which foods are best for you.

FLUIDS

 • What is the best fluid to keep my child athlete hydrated?
Plain cold water is the best and most economical source of fluid. Cold fluids are absorbed faster than warm ones, and drinking water is the easiest way to rehydrate the body. It is a good idea to provide your child with his or her own water bottle.

 What is all the controversy about sports drinks?
Water is the best fluid to hydrate the child for practices and events lasting up to 90 minutes. If your child participates in long or all-day events, sports drinks or diluted fruit juices may be beneficial for carbohydrate replacement. The rule of thumb is 6% to 8% carbohydrate fluids; this means half-strength fruit juice, half-strength lemonade, and most sports drinks.

 How much fluid does it take to keep my child hydrated during sports events?
The child should be weighed before and after the exercising period to know how much fluid he or she lost. Then follow these basic guidelines to be sure your child is drinking enough because thirst is NOT an adequate indicator of the need for fluids.

BEFORE EXERCISE
Drink 10–14 ounces of cold water 1–2 hours before the activity.
Drink 10 ounces of cold water 10–15 minutes before the activity.

DURING EXERCISE
Drink 3–4 ounces of cold water every 15 minutes.

AFTER EXERCISE
Drink 2 cups (16 ounces) of cold water for every pound of weight loss.

Lemonade Thirst Quencher

DURING EXERCISE

a 6% carbohydrate solution
4 scoops of powdered lemonade drink mix per gallon of water

Nutrition Info per 8-ounce serving
Calories: 51
Carbohydrate: 13.4 (100%)

AFTER EXERCISE

a 12% carbohydrate solution
8 scoops of powdered lemonade drink mix per gallon of water

Nutrition Info per 8-ounce serving
Calories: 102
Carbohydrate: 26.9 (100%)

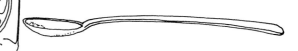

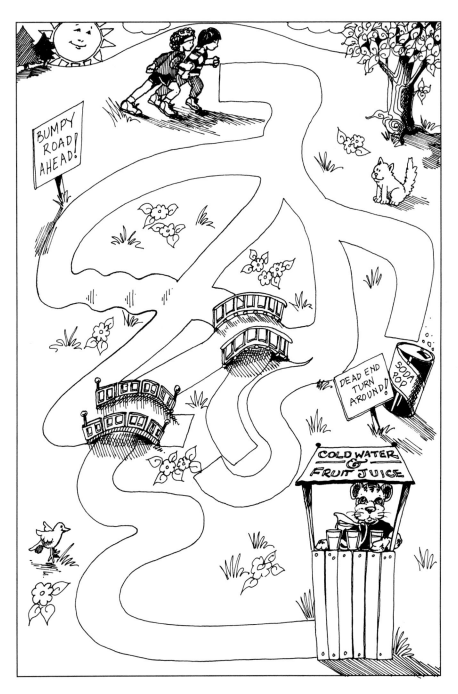

Exercising is thirsty work! Fluid is the most
important part of an athlete's diet.
Find the fastest route to the Tiger's
water and fruit juice stand.

EAT TO COMPETE

 • There's a lot of talk about pre-event eating. What are the best pre-event foods for my child athlete?

The pre-event meal serves two purposes;
1. to prevent the child from feeling hungry
2. to help supply fuel to the muscles during training and competition.

EAT	AVOID
complex carbohydrates	fat
water	protein
moderate portions	fiber
	last minute sweets

 • Does it matter when my child eats this pre-event meal?

Yes, it is best for your child to eat 3–4 hours before competition time. Your child may not feel well exercising with a full stomach. Some foods digest and leave the stomach quicker than others.

Fat	4–5 hours
Protein	3–4 hours
Carbohydrate	2–3 hours; *but remember, carbohydrate foods that are high in fiber may take longer.*

 • My child seems to have no appetite after hard training. Is it important that he or she eats immediately after the sports event?

The body is most receptive to replacing muscle carbohydrate, called glycogen, during the first 2 hours after hard exercise. It may be easier for your child to drink the carbohydrate rather than eat it. If this is the case, fruit juice or lemonade may be the answer. Sports drinks would be another choice, but most contain less carbohydrate than juice, and at this point, more is better. It is a good plan for the child to eat a high-carbohydrate MEAL within 5 hours after the event. There are a few suggestions below.

1 large baked potato with grated low-fat cheese and plain low-fat yogurt	2 cups spaghetti
Carrot sticks	⅔ cup meat sauce with mushrooms and peppers
1 cup fruit salad	2 pieces French bread
1 cup low-fat milk	1 cup sherbet
	1 cup low-fat milk

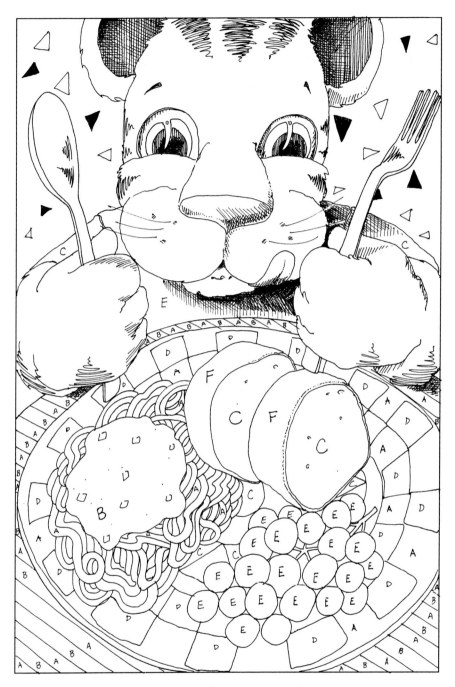

Color the puzzle to find out what Tiger eats before the big event. Use the color key below to choose your colors.

A white   **C** yellow   **E** purple

B red   **D** blue   **F** brown

GOOD FOOD FAST

Q: My family eats out two to three times each week. How can I make sure my child gets nutritious foods?

Good news; in the past few years, fast-food franchises and family-style restaurants have taken healthful eating more seriously and have added more low-fat, nutritious foods to their menus. The traffic lights below will help you and your child make informed food choices.

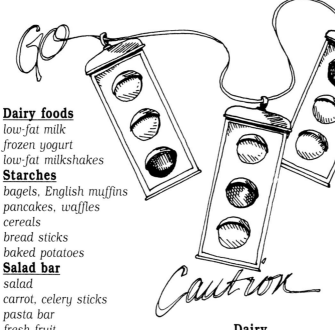

GO

Dairy foods
low-fat milk
frozen yogurt
low-fat milkshakes
Starches
bagels, English muffins
pancakes, waffles
cereals
bread sticks
baked potatoes
Salad bar
salad
carrot, celery sticks
pasta bar
fresh fruit
soups, not cream-based
low-fat dressings
Meats/main dishes
chicken filet
grilled chicken sandwich
chili with beans
plain hamburgers
vegetable pizza
chicken/turkey/ham/roast
beef sandwich or sub
Beverages
fruit, vegetable juices
lemonade
low-fat milk
Sauces
catsup
mustard
barbecue sauce

Caution

Dairy
2% milk
soft-serve ice cream
milkshakes
Starches
small order French fries
cornbread
Salad bar
chicken, tuna salad
coleslaw
macaroni/potato salad
cream-based soups
Meats/main dishes
cheeseburgers
steak sandwiches
cheese pizza
Beverages
diet soda
2% milk

Stop *(think again!)*

Dairy
whole milk
hard ice cream
Starches
biscuit, croissant
large order French fries
curly, cheese or other fries
pastry, pie or brownie
Salad bar
croutons
bacon bits
more than 2 tbsp of dressing
Meats/main dishes
fried chicken
fried chicken sandwich
fried fish/fried fish sandwich
fish or chicken nuggets
"super," "deluxe," or
"supreme" sandwich or burger
sausage, pepperoni or
extra cheese pizza
bacon burger
breakfast biscuits (egg
with sausage or steak)
sausage, bacon
Beverages
regular soda
whole milk
Sauces
mayonnaise
mayo-type sauces
alfredo sauce
hollandaise sauce
added butter or margarine

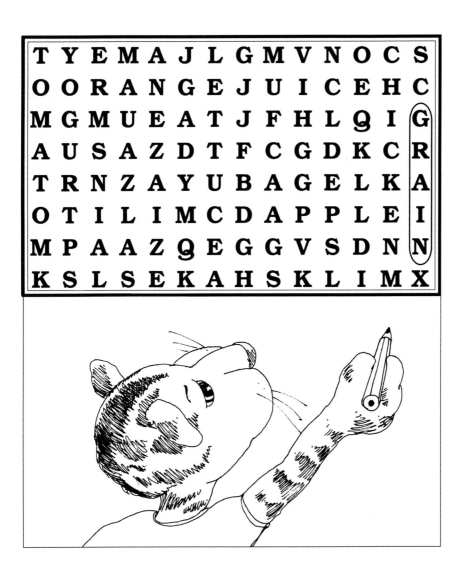

```
T Y E M A J L G M V N O C S
O O R A N G E J U I C E H C
M G M U E A T J F H L Q I G
A U S A Z D T F C G D K C R
T R N Z A Y U B A G E L K A
O T I L I M C D A P P L E I
M P A A Z Q E G G V S D N N
K S L S E K A H S K L I M X
```

Search and find the fast-food choices below that fit into a healthful sports diet (search only for **bold print words**). Remember, the words can be found across, up and down, diagonally and backward.

BREAKFAST	LUNCH	SNACK	DINNER
English **muffin**	**chicken** sandwich	frozen **yogurt**	cheese **pizza**
strawberry **jam**	multi**grain** bun	muffin (bran,	(thick crust
scrambled **egg**	**lettuce**	blueberry, etc)	with veggies)
orange juice	**tomato**	or **bagel**	side **salad**
milk	low-fat **milkshake**		**milk**
	apple brought from home		

THE WEIGHT BALANCE

 • How do I know if my child is overweight, underweight or at • just the right weight?

There is NO one specific weight that is perfect for your child. Pediatricians and registered dietitians assess the child's weight by using national standards based on age and sex. There is an acceptable weight RANGE for each increment of height of the child.

 •Everyone says my child will "grow into his or her weight." •Is this true?

It is normal for your child to add extra body fat in preparation for the "growth spurt." But, if you are concerned about your child's weight, you may seek the advice of a pediatrician and a registered dietitian who can determine your child's growth potential and make recommendations for a healthy weight.

 • My child has irregular eating habits and loves junk food. • Should he or she be on a diet?

The childhood years are none too early to learn a prudent, heart-healthy life-style. Encourage your child to eat foods low in "bad" fats, high in complex carbohydrates like whole-grain breads, fruits, vegetables, and low-fat dairy products; to eat foods high in dietary fiber; and to avoid excessive salt in the diet. Daily physical activity is another heart healthy life-style habit that will allow your child never to worry about the "D" word: diet. Parents need to be role models to teach kids that physical activity and healthful eating can be fun.

Recipes

SNACKS FOR THE OVERWEIGHT ATHLETE . . .
FAT-FREE BANANA MUFFINS

3 large well-ripened,
   mashed bananas
2 egg whites   } mix
⅓ cup nonfat milk

combine {
   ⅓ cup sugar
   1 tsp salt
   1 tsp baking soda
   ½ tsp baking powder
   ¾ cup whole-wheat flour
   ¾ cup plain white flour

SNACKS FOR THE UNDERWEIGHT ATHLETE . . .
OLD FASHIONED BANANA MUFFINS

3 large well-ripened bananas
1 egg
2 tbsp canola oil   } mix
⅓ cup low-fat milk (2% fat)

combine {
   ½ cup sugar
   1 tsp salt
   1 tsp baking soda
   ½ tsp baking powder
   ¾ cup whole-wheat flour
   ¾ cup plain white flour

TO MIX FOR BOTH RECIPES: Stir wet and dry mixtures together until moistened and lumpy. Fill cups of a muffin tin sprayed with vegetable spray ⅔ full, and bake at 350°F for 25 minutes or until toothpick inserted into muffin comes out clean. Recipe serves 12.

Nutrition Info: Fat-Free: Calories: 106   protein: 2.9 g (11%)   carbohydrate: 24.0 g (86%)   fat: 0.4 g (3%)
            Old Fashioned: Calories: 142   protein: 2.9 g (8%)   carbohydrate: 26.8 g (73%)   fat: 3.2 g (19%)

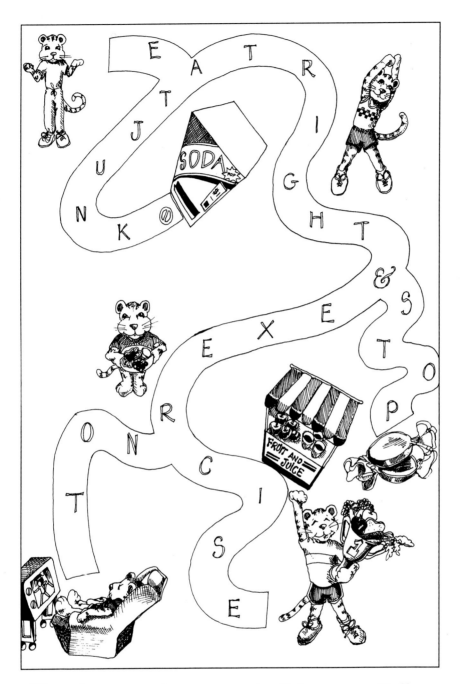

There's a secret message in this maze. Follow the path to a healthy life-style and spell out an important message along the way.

_____ _____ __

_____